work out your abs

For my wife, Chiara, and my daughters, Elisa and Francesca

Special thanks to Valentina Volpe, Cristina Canova, and
Linda Perina, who kindly posed for the photographs.

This book was written for people who want to maintain and improve their health
and fitness using abdominal exercises. Each reader must take personal responsibili-
ty for deciding to what extent the exercises recommended by the author are appropriate. The choice of program depends on the fitness level and health of the individual. If you are not sure what your status is, or if you are working out for thera-
peutic purposes, seek the approval of your physician or physical therapist before
starting the program.

English translation by Paolo Landi; translation edited by Isabel Stein.

Library of Congress Cataloging-in-Publication Data Available

10 9 8 7 6 5 4 3 2 1

Published by Sterling Publishing Company, Inc.
387 Park Avenue South, New York, N.Y. 10016
First published in Italy and ©1999 by DEMETRA S.r.l.
under the title *L'"arte" degli Addominali*
English translation ©2002 by Sterling Publishing Co., Inc.,
licensed by Demetra S.r.l.
Distributed in Canada by Sterling Publishing
c/o Canadian Manda Group, One Atlantic Avenue, Suite 105
Toronto, Ontario, Canada M6K 3E7
Distributed in Great Britain and Europe by Cassell PLC
Wellington House, 125 Strand, London WC2R 0BB, England
Distributed in Australia by Capricorn Link (Australia) Pty. Ltd.
P.O. Box 704, Windsor, NSW 2756 Australia

Sterling ISBN 0-8069-7891-0

work out
your abs

Roberto Maccadanza

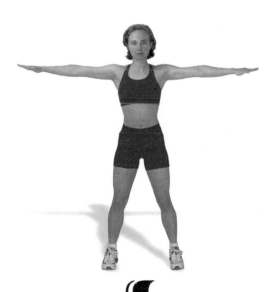

Sterling Publishing Co., Inc.
New York

CONTENTS

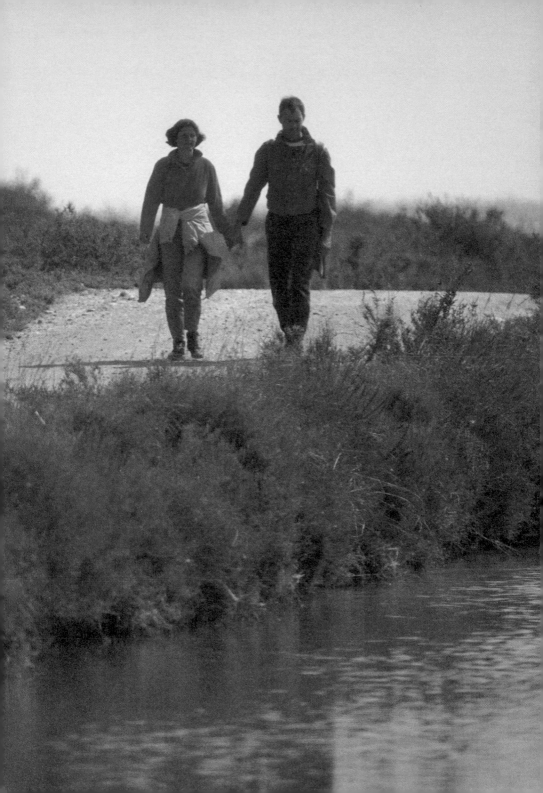

THE BODY AND MOVEMENT

WHY EXERCISE?

At times we may be gripped by a sudden urge to join the same gym as our girlfriend or boyfriend. We start off with the best of intentions, and after a couple of sessions, we find any excuse to avoid going back, instead buying that attractive piece of equipment recommended by a neighbor, for whom it solved all problems. A week or two after being welcomed into the home, the infernal equipment has become an unwanted guest, to the point that we will go to any lengths to avoid even looking at it. We come to philosophical conclusions about the routine of daily living – which is always the same regardless of physical activity, exhaustion and sweat – and so there is no reason to even let it concern us.

We will try to answer the question that opens this chapter in such a way that even the most confirmed critic of physical exercise will have a definite change of heart.

The human body was created for the functions of movement and inactivity, rest and flight. Over time, as a result of technological advances, there is less and less need to move because cars and elevators – not to mention the use of computers – and the Internet – have caused motor activity to give way to inertia.

Society itself does not encourage movement; the scarcity of open spaces where children can play and adults can move freely, devoting some time to their bodies, is unfortunately a common condition in our cities.

However, our bodies need to be stimulated if we want to keep them in good shape. Routine daily activities (getting up, walking, shopping, etc.) are not enough in themselves to stimulate the body. This is why it's necessary to plan activities based on physical exercise, which will allow our bodies to adapt to the kinds of movements that in the long run will be beneficial.

FUNCTIONAL EFFECTS OF MOVEMENT

To fully understand the importance of physical exercise, it is essential to explain the effects derived from it. These effects will be subdivided for our ease of understanding, but keep in mind that when the body reacts to the stimulus of exercise, it does so in its entirety, both physically and psychologically, and not in a compartmentalized way.

Having noted that, we will analyze in detail the principal effects of physical exercise on:
- The skeletal system
- The muscular system
- Joints
- The respiratory system
- The circulatory system
- The digestive system
- The nervous system
- Psychological and social well-being.

▶ **Skeletal system**. Movement stimulates bone growth both in length and width, especially during the early years of life. With exercise, the bones will be nourished better and consequently will become stronger and more resilient, combating possible trauma more effectively.

▶ **Muscular system**. Exercise causes significant changes in the muscles: esthetically it changes their appearance, and it can make them work more economically, giving them flexibility and stamina. Muscles increase their mass through growth in the number of fibers and capillaries and, by increasing their nutritional reserve, they can work better and longer.

▶ **Joints**. Exercise has an effect on the joints and their components (ligaments, capsules, and articular areas), making them more efficient. More synovial fluid (the substance inside the joints which allows for fluidity of motion) is produced, thus improving movement, making the ligaments more elastic and resilient, and therefore also reinforcing the membrane covering the joints.

▶ **Respiratory system**. Because its function, along with the cardiovascular system, is to supply oxygen, the respiratory system increases its activities considerably during movement. The intensity of respiratory actions, the functionality of the organs directly involved (lungs, bronchi, alveoli), and the mobility of the thoracic (chest) cavity and the spinal column all increase, with a resulting improvement in thoracic position.

WHY A BOOK ON THE ABDOMINAL MUSCLES?

Why indeed? Such a question is understandable if we recall that we have often heard it said that the body should be considered as a whole, so to consider only one part of it would seem limited.

Here is a concise but valid explanation, which will become clearer as you read the book.

We focus on the abdominal muscles because:

- They serve important functions in the resting state and dynamics of the human body;

- It is easy to make mistakes if we do incorrect exercises and are unaware of the underlying theory;

- Abdominals can be a starting point in reawakening the desire to listen to our own bodies and their needs;

- We won't have to put that last pair of pants or last skirt from "when we were in shape" in mothballs.

Everything revolves around a willingness to work on yourself, to feel good about yourself, and to ensure that physical exercise becomes a healthy daily habit.

▶ Circulatory system. A closed system made up of specialized structures (veins, arteries, and capillaries), the focal point of which is the heart. The heart supplies the push necessary to allow blood to reach all the different parts of the body requiring energy, especially during physical exercise. The heart reacts in two ways to physical activity: by increasing heartbeat rate and by increasing heart contraction power. Increasing heartbeat rate is not an economical reaction, because the heart does not have time to completely refill itself and therefore puts into circulation a smaller amount of blood. Such a situation is typical of out-of-shape people. Cardiac output increase, on the other hand, is a functional reaction, because, since the heart is forced to work less, it is able to pump more blood with each contraction. Regular physical exercise will produce a variation of the second kind of reaction, much more important from a sports point of view and for preventing cardiac problems which may arise as we age.

▶ **Digestive system**. Movement improves the digestion and elimination processes, making the functions of the stomach, intestines, and liver more effi-

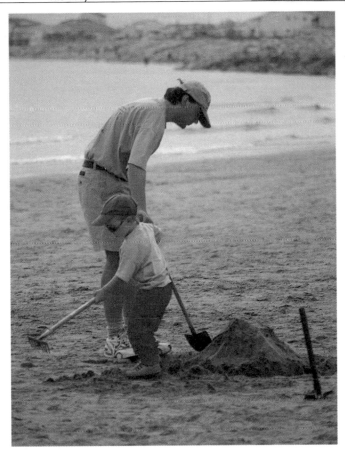

There are other ways of getting exercise besides sports.

cient. The liver performs extremely important functions for the development of motor activity: conversion of sugar into glycogen, conversion of lactic acid (a waste product of muscular activity) into glycogen, and control of the venous flow to the heart.

▶ **Nervous system**. The changes produced by physical exercise tend to improve the quality of motion, making it more precise, coordinated, and fast-paced and therefore more economical and complete. We acquire some automatic capabilities which prove to be very important, especially for sports, with significant improvement in reaction times and sensory abilities (hearing, vision, touch, and balance).

▶ **Psychological and social consequences**. A strong correlation exists between motor activity and mental activity, and much teaching is based on this concept, from the basic level on.

The relationship between intellectual development and movement is a very close one, starting in early infancy, and movement influences imagination, receptivity, and memory.

Even though we may tend to think otherwise, motor activity increases intellectual performance, improving mental flexibility and response to stimuli. The solution to motor problems simply transforms an act of the intellect into motion. Not only are states of emotion (joy, happiness, sadness, and tension) thus stimulated, but also control over them, which allows us to exert better balance and greater self-control, even in everyday life.

Thanks to motor activity, a sense of self-esteem, self-awareness, and self-worth – qualities not to be underestimated – may blossom anew, especially in the later years, a time which otherwise might be far from stimulating.

THE RIGHT APPROACH

The main problem is discovering how to approach working on your body to get positive results.

It would be very simple to let yourself be seduced by a product promising to get you back in shape with very little work, or to take a "magic" pill that supposedly will solve the problem in a flash.

Working on yourself is not easy and calls for a major commitment, interest, and involvement.

▶ The best methods of getting results from working on your body are these three:
- Go to the gym and be coached by a qualified staff member;
- Be coached at home by a personal trainer;
- Make use of outside aids (equipment, books, etc.).

In all these situations, there is the possibility of designing a workout plan based on your individual potential and desired goals – in simple terms, creating a personalized workout. The first two options are definitely recommended, but are not always doable.

▶ The concept of a **personalized workout** is essential if you want to avoid the following situations:
- Leaving the gym after two lessons;
- Spending a lot of money without accomplishing a thing;
- Losing interest if the goals prove to be beyond your grasp.

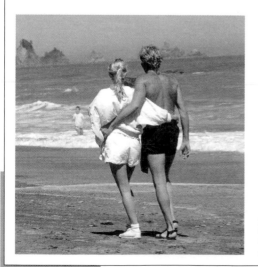

Paying attention to ourselves and regaining personal balance by working on our bodies improves self-perception and allows us to live well with ourselves and with others.

THE ABDOMINAL MUSCLES

When talking about abs, the first thought is of those glossy images in the press of good-looking young men and alluring girls showing off flat, almost sculpted and very appealing tummies, symbolizing (outwardly only) physical fitness and esthetic beauty, images of bodies reminiscent of Greek gods, unrealistic representations of men and women.

People have an overwhelming desire to look just like these models at any cost, without taking into consideration individual structural differences or what goes on inside their own bodies. What's important is what shows on the outside; at least that's the recipe for success in our society. The problem is made clear when we realize that the goal of those images is unattainable, and therefore, in reaction, we decide to do absolutely nothing more, with obvious consequences, as we look for the easy justification that we're past the right age. To think that taking care of oneself is the prerogative of the young and that it is beyond our own daily routines is surely a mistake. The abs are parts of our bodies that need attention not only during particularly favorable situations in our lives (adolescence, youth), but also during pregnancy, middle age, and beyond.

As a matter of fact, anyone who thinks that middle age must bring with it a protruding stomach, annoying padding of fat around the hips, and a flabby paunch makes a very big mistake!

Seeing only what is visible on the outside without taking into consideration that the body needs to be evaluated as a whole is a basic error. We need to look at the warning sign of a paunch not as a demand for prolonged sessions at the gym or rivers of sweat poured over some infernal piece of equipment, but as the body calling for salvation, assistance, and help in reclaiming that past sense of well-being, now long forgotten.

In practice, what is it that makes us realize that the time has come to take serious steps and that the situation may be getting out of hand?

As with any respectable personal program, the starting point must be an evaluation of your own state of physical fitness, and in particular the abs, using the information to determine the most appropriate steps to be taken.

Even though our attention is directed to the structure of the abdominal muscles – for which a very specific self-examination is given in the following pages – it is important to have an overall view of your own physical condition. This allows a better workout organization and, more importantly, avoids running into situations that, if we ignore them, can cause problems later.

> It will be important to evaluate:
> - Your overall state of health, perhaps having your physician give you a checkup to provide a picture of your cardiorespiratory functioning;
> - Your diet (see pages 99 to 107);
> - Your personal strength and resistance levels.

All of this may seem very complicated and at first glance even scary, because it might look like a workout program for assault troops.... But take note: In some cases working on your body might very well be a highly strategic undertaking.

WHERE ARE YOU?

Here are some suggestions for self-evaluation of your fitness.

▶ To get an idea of your cardiovascular capacity, find a route of approximately one kilometer (about 0.6 mile) — for example, a walk around your neighborhood — which can be done in about 15 to 20 minutes, walking at a normal pace. Before starting, measure your heart rate, writing it down on a piece of paper. At the end of the walk, check your rate again, and then check it after one minute. If the third heart rate measure exceeds the first, resting one, it means that special care should be paid during workout to

Gently place the tips of your index and middle fingers in two different places: A) on the side of the trachea to measure carotid arterial rate (the pulse); B) on the wrist of the opposite arm, below the base of the thumb, to measure the radial arterial rate (pulse).

what is called warming up (see page 50). When you repeat the measurements after one month of the program, the heart rate values should get closer.

▶ To evaluate arm strength, perform the following test.
Put yourself in the position shown in the photograph (facing page, top) and lower your body, bending your arms (bottom photo) until they are parallel to the floor. Count how many push-ups you are able to do in one minute. If you count fewer than 5 and you feel achy all over, it means your arms are at best strong enough to lift a ball-point pen.

WHAT BODY TYPE ARE YOU?

If we wanted to reduce everything to a mere analysis of the abdominal area, we would make a mistake for sure.
Your body cannot be seen as an assembly of different parts, separate from one another, separate entities to be worked on, but as a whole unit working in concert. To better understand how to work on your body, let's do a brief survey of the main body types, which each one of us can easily understand.

▶ **Endomorph**. Characterized by an overall rounded and soft body with very limited muscle mass.
Such an individual has fairly ample and rounded stomach and buttocks, with high shoulders and a developed chest, has the tendency to accumulate fat, and is large-boned. In women with this body type, the pelvis is broader than the shoulders.

▶ **Mesomorph**. Characterized by a strong muscle mass; large breastbone, hips, and shoulders; and a well developed chest. There is a tendency to be muscular and the shoulders are broader than the pelvis.

types we fall in order to see what can be expected of us, without dreaming of looking like an actor, a wonderful athlete, or a gorgeous top model.
If after the self-evaluation you have the idea that your body is asking for help be-

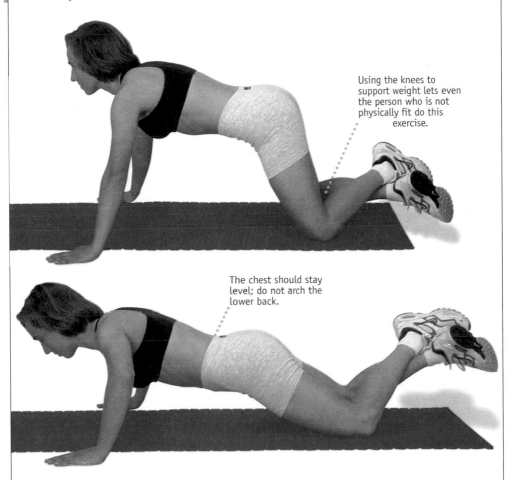

Using the knees to support weight lets even the person who is not physically fit do this exercise.

The chest should stay level; do not arch the lower back.

▶ **Ectomorph**. Characterized by a fragile and delicate structure with long bones, long neck and limbs, and without good muscle mass, therefore a flat stomach and buttocks. Shoulders and pelvis are of equal breadth.
Each of us should try to identify into which classification of the above body

fore you have serious problems, it is time to get to work!
We hope you will exercise and avoid becoming someone who, because of profound imbalances in the abdominal musculature, finds himself or herself disadvantaged, both physically and psychologically, for example, the following:

- People with relaxed and swollen stomachs (**A**);
- Very tall people with overly curved backs (lumbar hyperlordosis, **B**);
- Elderly people in poor health who need a cane (**C**).

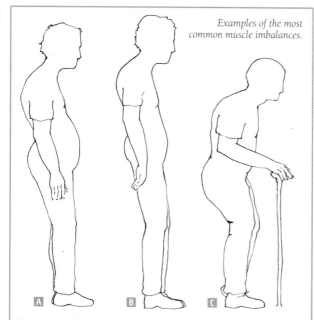

Examples of the most common muscle imbalances.

WHY WE GET PAUNCHES

Let's clarify the causes that may determine what is commonly called a paunch, because such a condition does not always depend on abdominal structure problems, although in the majority of cases this does play a fundamental role.

There can be several sources, including:

- Muscular
- Dietary
- Age and gender
- Special situations (postpartum, forced inactivity)
- Muscular imbalances.

Let's analyze these various causes in detail.

▶ **Muscular causes**. Reduced movement, also called hypokinesis, is a typical scenario in our daily lives, where cars, escalators, and elevators take the place of the human body and its potential, causing the whole muscular system, and in particular the abdominal area, to lack tone and vitality.

Such a condition can be easily found in many everyday situations: the person forced to spend a great deal of the day inside a car (traveling salesman, truck driver) or in a static position (clerk), the child sitting in front of television for hours on end, or the teenager at the computer – even the older person who, thinking himself no longer able to do anything, including working, stops moving, with terrible consequences for his fitness.

▶ **Dietary causes**. A poorly balanced diet, less time devoted to meals and mealtime skipped altogether, plus digestive difficulties linked to emotional or physical stress may create situations which, while not directly affecting abdominal structure, nevertheless have significant influence in the personal sphere and on the predisposition to physical effort.

▶ **Age and gender**. The relationship between an individual's age and gender at various stages of life may be the source of particular problems. For example, the higher percentage of body fat in women than in men, its localization in specific

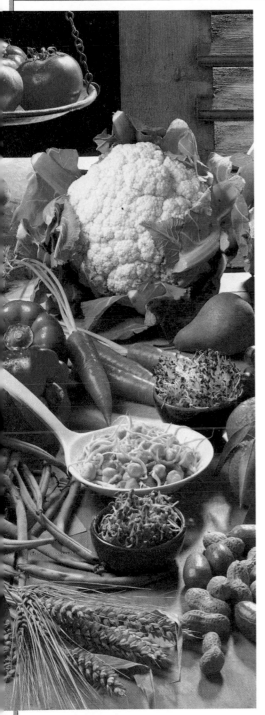

areas (buttocks, abdomen, hips), can create a feeling of heaviness in the central part of the body, which may be accentuated during menopause, a time in which a woman's physical and psychological situation may reduce her sense of being in optimal shape.

When it comes to old age, possible physiological problems of decreased flexibility of the spinal column, the reduction in respiratory capacity and, not least, an emotional state linked to a feeling of uselessness that many elderly people have certainly do not contribute to the maintenance of a good level of physical exercise.

▶ **Special situations**. The time after childbirth is an extremely important period in a woman's life, but at the same time one that may be very problematic as well, especially because of the functional recovery it requires.

Such a period assumes a restoration to optimal conditions, primarily involving the abdominal muscles which, after proving how elastic they can be, have to return in short time to functioning well.

Forced inactivity resulting from a variety of causes such as accidents or other pathologies has an influence on a person's overall condition, including abdominal muscle structure.

▶ **Muscular imbalances**. Finally, it should be noted that an imbalance, for example between weak abdominals and overly toned back muscles, may favor the onset of a paunch. This condition may be found in the sports environment, with athletes who, although appearing to be in good physical shape, may have thigh and upper back muscles that are too strong and may find themselves in a state of imbalance, which in time could cause problems.

ABDOMINAL MUSCLES: PURPOSE AND FUNCTION

When we think about abdominal muscles, our minds turn to the simple concept of the belly, but these muscles should be viewed in terms of the general balance of the body in its entirety. The abs work for the containment and protection of the internal organs, thus creating, together with the pelvic structure, a very important and efficient defense mechanism. The containment function is crucial in particular situations such as pregnancy, a condition that also demonstrates the elasticity of this muscle structure. Abs work for the preservation of body balance both at rest and in motion, offering their contribution to maintaining correct posture in synergy with other muscle groups. The fundamental function of the abs is to support body positioning during movement. They represent the juncture between pelvis and torso, thus assuring efficient movement of the lower limbs. By securing the rib cage to the pelvis, they provide solid support for upper limb movement. At work, they are in opposition to the back muscles, thus protecting torso stability during all movement. For this reason, they are essential in preventing lumbago, that annoying lumbar back pain affecting many people, which can result in temporary or permanent disability.

ABDOMINAL MUSCLES AND THE SPINAL COLUMN

To insure the stability and posture of the spinal column, it is important to make some observations on the relationship between the two structures. The spinal column performs some very important functions: in addition to supporting the torso, it protects the spinal cord contained inside the spinal column from impacts and wounds. It is formed by the joining of 33 or 34 short bones called vertebrae, arranged vertically one atop the other. Vertebrae are separated from one another by intervertebral disks and held together by ligaments covering the entire column.

Because of the area they occupy and their function, vertebrae are divided as follows: cervical, thoracic, lumbar, sacral, and coccygeal.

Viewed from the front, the spinal column is straight, but viewed from the side it shows characteristic linked curvatures, some that are mobile (the cervical and lumbar sections) and some of semi-rigid or rigid structure (thoracic, sacral, and coccygeal).

▶ We will see later how some abdominal muscles (transverse, internal oblique, iliopsoas, and quadratus

From top to bottom, the spinal (vertebral) column consists of 7 cervical vertebrae, 12 thoracic vertebrae, 5 lumbar vertebrae, 5 fused sacral vertebrae, and 4 or 5 fused coccygeal vertebrae that form the coccyx. The spinal column has a cervical curve, a thoracic curve, and a lumbar curve.

Facing page: Illu. A shows the correct position of the spinal column in the stance. Illustration B shows an incorrect position (asthenic or weak), which has a tendency to accentuate the cervical, thoracic, and lumbar curvatures.

lumborum) attach to the lumbar section of the spinal column and therefore play a primary role in pelvic stasis and dynamics, along with some spinal muscles and some muscles of the lower limbs.

In the asthenic (weak) position, a condition readily found in many people with relaxed posture, relaxation accentuates the spinal curvatures (**B**): there is lumbar hyperlordosis and increased lumbar kyphosis (backward curvature), and cervical lordosis (lordosis=forward curvature). The pelvis is rotated backwards, a condition aggravated by the iliopsoas muscles' work, which tends to increase such position. A similar condition is noted in the late stages of pregnancy.

The most important role in correcting lumbar hyperlordosis is played by the rectus abdominis muscle. In fact it is sufficient to contract the buttocks and rectus abdominis to straighten lumbar lordosis. Therefore, it can be said that the abdominal muscles play a role in the conscious straightening of lumbar lordosis and thus in correct spinal column positioning (**A**).

HOW A MUSCLE WORKS

We have already seen the structural importance of the abdominal musculature and what problems can arise if it is not stimulated to movement. Now it is important to define how a muscle works in order to best determine its type of action during exercise.

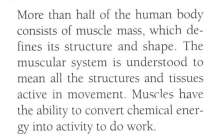
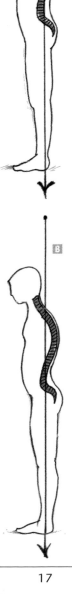

More than half of the human body consists of muscle mass, which defines its structure and shape. The muscular system is understood to mean all the structures and tissues active in movement. Muscles have the ability to convert chemical energy into activity to do work.

▶ The human body is made up of nearly 455 muscles, having specialized structures and functions in relation to their type (striated, smooth, voluntary, involuntary, etc.). A muscle is formed by the combination of elongated bands of muscle fiber which attach to the bones by means of tendons, fibrous cords that create points of support for the contractible muscle structures, which, in contracting and releasing, give rise to movement involving not only the particular muscle, but the entire organism.

▶ Muscles can become excessively enlarged in mass (hypertrophy), in which case we see an increase in strength along with an increase in their diameters. Each time the brain sends a nerve impulse, a section of the muscle fibers contracts, changing both shape and length and determining movement by means of the tendons. When the order that the nerve transmitted has been carried out, the muscle fibers return to their initial length. The more a muscle is used, the greater the amount of fiber will be in play; by continually being exercised, fibers increase in thickness. As a consequence, the muscle develops, increasing its volume and strength.

It is important not to keep muscles contracted between one exercise and the next in order to avoid hardening of the muscles, which eventually will run the risk of becoming ugly and nonfunctional.

To get good results, it is necessary to work against resistance – that is, engage the muscle in greater and greater workloads. Two other changes to the muscle in motion can be noted, related to the increase in capillaries: its improved working condition (elimination of waste products and better supply of oxygen) and improved biochemistry (better utilization of the sources of energy inside the muscle).

SOURCES OF ENERGY FOR MUSCLE WORK

In order to do its job, a muscle needs energy, measurable in calories, which it gets from food.

The substances supplying energy are classified as: **sugars** and **fats**, the two most important, and **proteins**, whose main job is to rebuild cells that have been destroyed. Proteins can be converted into energy only in the absence of the first two substances. The muscle absorbs the sugars (more precisely, the carbohydrates), which are converted immediately into energy, and fats, in a longer process.

The real energy reserves are made up by fats, which as they accumulate form adipose tissue, the cause of many problems from an esthetic and functional point of view, but which muscular work can eliminate over time. Muscle work also produces waste products (lactic acid), which as they accumulate create a feeling of fatigue and heat (to combat the cold of winter, we rub our cold hands together). The energy necessary to support life (the so-called basal metabolism) is on average 1500 calories per day, which are burned both in performing any kind of activity as well as in complete stasis, simply by the body's carrying out its vital functions (digestion, maintaining body temperature, respiration, cardiac contractions, etc.).

About half the body is made up of muscle mass, which determines its structure and shape. This illustration shows the principal muscles of the human body.

PROGRESSIVE OVERLOAD

Milo of Crotona, a Greek athlete in the 6th century B.C., used to lift a small calf every day from the day of its birth. Each day the calf got bigger, so the man grew stronger and more powerful. When the calf became a bull, Milo was still able to perform his daily routine.

Such a story contains a valid explanation of the principle of progressive overload and an effective plan for achieving it.

Progressive overload is the basis of the workout program you will undertake and is a main component in training, since it is based on the physiological law of adaptability. Muscle, just like bone of the skeletal structure, follows the principle that necessity creates ability – the more a structure is challenged, the more it is able to tolerate and adapt to the new condition. If bones, for example, are not used, they lose minerals, becoming lighter, more porous, and more fragile as a result (a very dangerous condition known as osteoporosis). When bones and muscles are used, a fitness effect results.

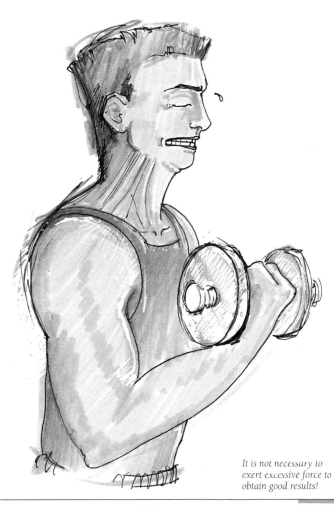

It is not necessary to exert excessive force to obtain good results!

19

We cannot talk about a fitness program if we limit ourselves to always doing the same number of exercises for an identical number of times. We have a program only when we apply the principle of progressive overload. There are many ways to introduce progressive overload.

▶ The riskiest system is to **increase the intensity** of exertion – that is, more hurried movements or lifting heavier weights.

▶ A safer method is **to increase the duration** of exertion, use a little more resistance, or carry the weight a little further.

▶ The most guaranteed method is **to increase the frequency** of the exertion: do it one additional time in the course of a week.

This last will be the method applied in our workout program, which each of you will implement based on how successful you were in the previous session.

CALORIES AND ENERGY EXPENDITURE

How many calories can be burned through physical exercise? Ironing, washing dishes, and rushing through household chores in one hour, for example, will burn 150 calories (a housewife covers approximately 3 to 4 miles per day staying home). Doing light morning exercise uses up almost 200 calories per hour. Climbing stairs burns 250 calories per hour, while swimming or playing tennis uses over 400 calories per hour. Considering that one gram of fat is equal to 9 calories, it is possible to calculate that in one month of daily morning activity about 400 grams (almost a pound) of fat can be lost. At first glance this doesn't look like much, but when added to other daily activities (climbing stairs, walking, moving about, etc.) and to some healthy revision of our eating habits, it is possible to expect results which are good both physically and psychologically. There is also the possibility of burning 400 calories in one hour playing tennis, chopping wood, or doing intensive sessions of a physical workout. But burning that many calories right away would be a titanic assignment for anybody just starting to do physical activity for the first time, particularly taking into account a possible lack of patience and total absence of training. The alternative therefore is plan to burn these calories throughout the day, doing specific movements involving the abs and making sure that the body is stimulated to move and to work harder and harder.

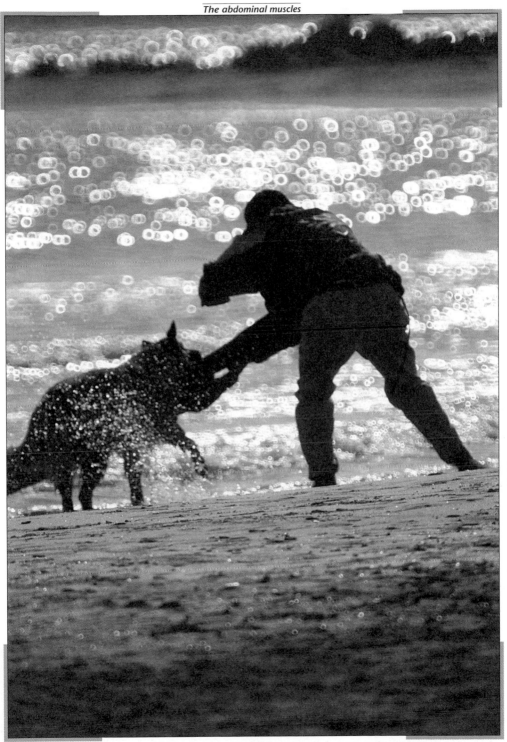

Abdominals and movement

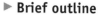

▶ Brief outline

As with the majority of our muscles, the abdominal muscles are symmetrical: they have the same structure and shape on the right side and the left side of the body.

At their point of juncture they are the source of a longitudinal fibrous septum (linea alba), in the middle of which is the navel.

The abdominal muscles are the **rectus abdominis**, **transverse** (transversus abdominis), **internal oblique**, **external oblique** (located in the front of the torso), and the **quadratus lumborum** and **iliopsoas** (located in the back of the torso).

As explanations of muscle function have clearly shown, the abdominal muscles come decisively into play in synergy with other muscles, letting us perform a wide variety of movements, from ones that are part of the simplest daily routine (e.g., getting out of bed in the morning, moving about while seated in the office chair, walking to go shopping, running to catch the bus) to ones that require greater effort (lifting a vase from the floor or performing a much more specialized sports activity such as throwing a javelin, executing a long jump, or playing volleyball).

Knowledge of the abdominal musculature from the anatomical and functional points of view will let you undertake the exercises knowing what area you are working and getting the maximum results from your exercise routine.

RECTUS ABDOMINIS MUSCLES

These form two muscular bands extending along the front of the abdomen, on either side of the midline. They are attached at the top of the 5th, 6th, and 7th

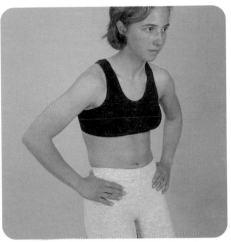

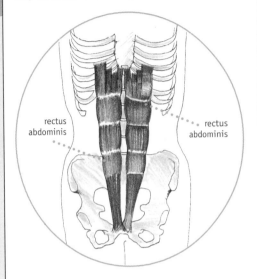

rectus abdominis — rectus abdominis

ribs, on the costal cartilage and on the xiphoid process (lower end of the sternum), and at the lower ends with a strong tendon that is attached to the upper edge of the pubis. The simultaneous contraction of the two rectus muscles causes a flexing of the chest and lowering of the rib cage at the same time.

TRANSVERSUS MUSCLES

The transversus muscles form the deepest level of the abdominal wall's broad muscles. They are inserted behind the xiphoid process in the midsection, passing under the rectus muscle to the muscle on the opposite side; the high ends are on the internal aspect of the last 6 ribs, and the low ends are on the upper edge of the pubic symphysis and the pubis. Simultaneous contraction gives rise to a narrowing of the abdominal cavity that pulls in the stomach. This plays a fundamental role in preventing ptosis (downward displacement) of the abdominal viscera.

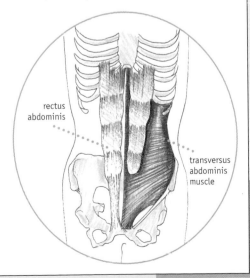

rectus abdominis

transversus abdominis muscle

23

INTERNAL OBLIQUE MUSCLE

Its upper ends insert on the cartilage of the last 3 or 4 ribs and on the xiphoid process (lower part of the sternum). The lower ends connect to the iliac crest. It joins in the middle with the contralateral muscle.

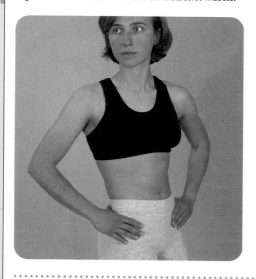

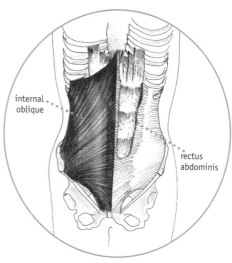

When the two muscles contract at the same time, the torso bends forward; if the action is unilateral, the torso will bend to that side.

EXTERNAL OBLIQUE MUSCLE

It is attached to the lower 7 ribs, the anterior edge of the iliac crest, the pubic bone, and the contralateral external oblique muscle. When contraction is on both sides, the torso will bend forward (helping the move-ment of the rectus abdominis); when the action is one-sided, there is a bending to the same side and, at the same time, a rotation of the opposite side.

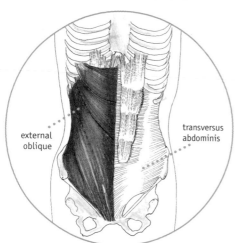

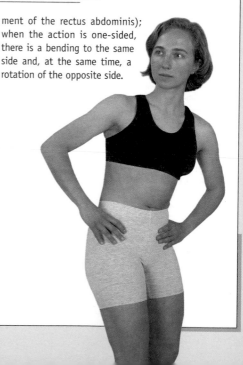

QUADRATUS LUMBORUM

The quadratus lumborum is part of the posterior abdominal musculature. This flat, square muscle attaches to the transverse process of the upper 4 lumbar vertebrae, on the twelfth rib, and on the inferior edge of the iliac crest. A bilateral contraction keeps the lumbar lordosis in a state of balance.

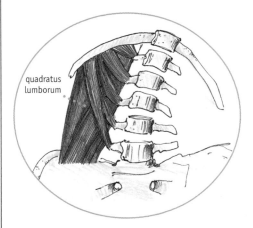

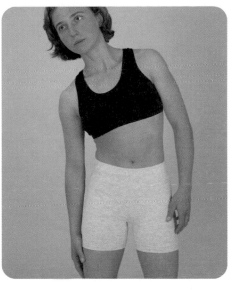

A unilateral contraction causes side bending.

ILIOPSOAS

This is made up of two muscles. The psoas attaches to the twelfth rib and all the lumbar vertebrae; the iliacus attaches to the pelvic bone. Both meet and attach by a single tendon to the beginning of the femur.

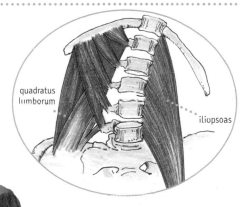

When the iliopsoas contracts, it becomes the most powerful flexor of the thigh, but also flexes the lumbar spine and the pelvis forward and downward. Keep this in mind; it could be the cause of problems if the exercises are done incorrectly.

This movement just shows the muscle action but should not be done, since it tends to arch the lumbar area.

25

Self-test of your abdominals

Finally we come to the part that interests us the most, namely, an evaluation of the abdominal muscles. The suggested self-examination is broken down into two parts. The first part consists of a few questions, which you must answer very truthfully; the second part has a few simple physical exercises which, during the program, will be our way of keeping track of the work being done.

► The suggested small tests (which you will use later on to check the fitness level of your abs), along with the answers you give to the questions below, should tell you about your need to get started.

► The self-evaluation exercises will be repeated at the beginning of the workout program, since they form not only the basis for the workout, but also a control measure allowing for evaluation at any time of the results achieved and of your state of fitness.

PLEASE ANSWER THESE QUESTIONS

► Do you get a feeling of exertion and heaviness when performing the simplest daily tasks (e.g., putting on shoes or lifting a weight from the floor), a feeling concentrated in your lower back and abdomen?

► Do you sometimes feel pain in your back?

► If you go to buy clothing, do you need to buy a larger size because your waist is rather large?

► If you pinch the flab on your stomach between your thumb and forefinger, does it exceed 3/4 inch (2 cm) in thickness?

► When summer comes, are you uncomfortable in a bathing suit?

► After eating, do you have a swollen stomach and an unpleasant feeling of heaviness?

► If you have to run to catch a bus, do you feel as if your stomach area weighs you down?

If you answered "yes" to more than one of the questions, your abs could be a problem and it is important to start resolving it.

LET'S TAKE A PRACTICAL TEST

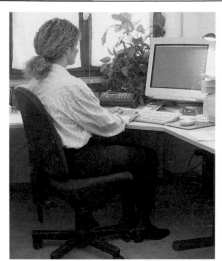

Find a little time to exercise, even at your desk.

1 Sit in a chair without leaning against the backrest and put your hands on your stomach; try to inhale and exhale, inflating and flattening your belly. Was it hard or easy to do?

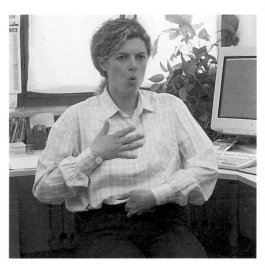

2 Still in the same position, exhale strongly through your mouth while pulling in your belly. With your fingers, try to feel whether your muscles are firming up or if they remain flaccid or flimsy.

3 Turn in the chair as shown below, put hands on belly, and bend your head forward, chin to chest. Breathing normally, move down 4 to 6 inches (10 to 15 cm), 25 to 30 degrees. Can you hold this position for 20 seconds without starting to quiver?

Keeping feet firmly on the floor, try during this exercise to move down until you can feel your belly muscles contracting.

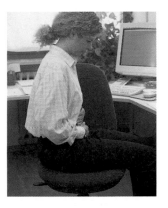

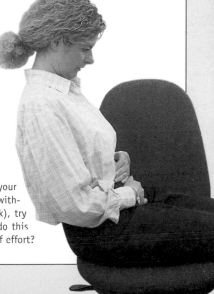

4 Find a heavy object to put your feet under (desk, cabinet, or your bed). With your hands behind the back of your neck, legs bent, without holding your breath (this will be explained later in the book), try to sit up until you can touch knees with your elbows. Can you do this 10 times in a row? If so, did you do it easily or did it take a lot of effort?

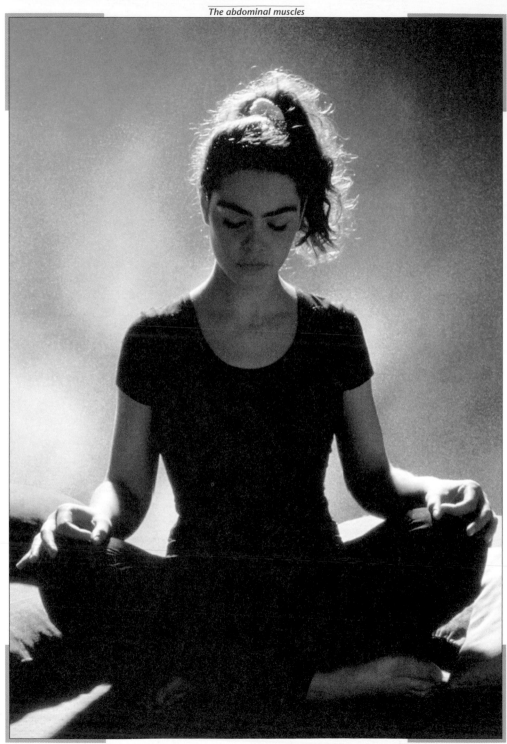

BREATHING

Breathing is a fundamental aspect of a workout aimed at improving abdominal muscle capacity. Breathing plays a very important role, mainly because it can prevent complex problems that might arise during incorrect execution of the exercises, as we will see in the following paragraphs.

The aim of breathing is to exchange gases between the body and the environment. The job of our breathing apparatus is to take oxygen into the body and let carbon dioxide out. The better this apparatus works, the better the effect on the body as a whole.

The main muscles involved in breathing are the diaphragm and intercostal muscles; by contracting and releasing, they let us inhale and exhale. The auxiliary muscles, which become involved only when deeper-than-normal breathing is called for, especially in exhaling, are the rectus abdominis, the internal and external obliques, and the quadratus lumborum (see pgs. 22 to 25).

Surely you have had the feeling that you

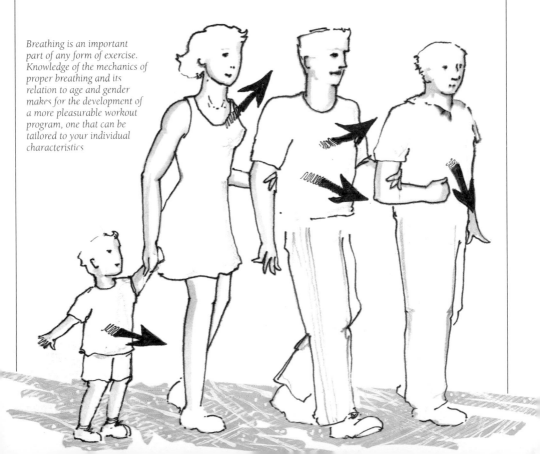

Breathing is an important part of any form of exercise. Knowledge of the mechanics of proper breathing and its relation to age and gender makes for the development of a more pleasurable workout program, one that can be tailored to your individual characteristics

need to take in more oxygen after prolonged physical effort (running to catch a bus for those who are less fit, or maybe a long workout session for the more athletic) and are panting, with your stomach moving rapidly in and out before returning to normal. The abdominal muscles are involved in conditions of labored breathing and in the return to normal conditions.

The breathing mechanism varies significantly in relation to age and gender.

► In **women**, breathing is of the upper costal (upper chest) type; the upper part of the respiratory structure is used. This distinctiveness becomes indispensable during pregnancy, when the presence of the fetus keeps the diaphragm from working appropriately.

from the above because of an increase in curvature of the thoracic spine (thoracic kyphosis) and muscular hypotonia (loss of original muscle tone). Mobility of the upper ribs is somewhat reduced and the upper lobe of the lung is no longer ventilated, and breathing becomes of the lower costal type, or even abdominal.

BREATHING AND BREATHING EXERCISES

One of the greatest errors in doing exercises for the abdominal muscles is expending as much effort as possible as intensely as possible, perhaps at the suggestion of a tough, muscular trainer. We re-

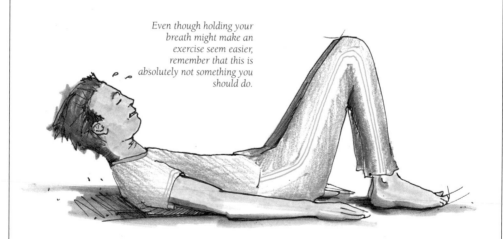

Even though holding your breath might make an exercise seem easier, remember that this is absolutely not something you should do.

► In **children**, breathing is of the abdominal (diaphragmatic) type.

► In **men**, it is of a mixed type, i.e., upper and lower costal (chest).

► In the **elderly**, breathing may vary

spond to this suggestion by trying to exert as much effort as possible, at the same time holding our breath, thus feeling that we could tolerate the strain better.

► Performing any exercise in a state of apnea (without breathing) can create excessive pressure in the chest, which will negatively affect coronary circulation, impeding correct heart function – all the more dangerous for those who are out of shape, elderly, or have heart problems.Such a condition can cause fainting, with uncontrolled increase in blood pressure. Using the proper breathing techniques while exercising will let you find the proper pace for your workout and give you a better idea of your physical strength. It will also restore to you that sense of wellbeing that may have been long forgotten because you do not do more physical exercise, and because of your hectic and stressful schedule. We should note that top-level athletes engaged in activities involving great muscle strength (weightlifters) tend to hold their breath during execution of their exercises to protect their spinal columns. Our program makes no pretense of reaching such a level of specialization; it will be necessary to check your breathing, as we will explain.

MOTIVATION

Motivation is very important in any kind of body work. Motivation allows for active participation in the workout regarding the mechanics of movement as well as its mental and psychological components. Within the framework of fitness programs, motivation must be the indispensable drive to achieving preestablished goals, and it becomes even more necessary if the program is not linked to a sports training regimen, but simply – and no less significantly – is for the benefit of your body and its everyday needs.

Motivation allows those with severe functional limitations to overcome these unfavorable conditions to whatever extent possible and get back to normal. Motivation has even greater value in the case of people who, though not in extremely grave condition, look forward to getting back to a stable situation. In our daily lives, the motivation towards movement is at very low levels. The search for stimuli that will force movement on us is diminished and limited by excessive use of cars, elevators, etc. and also by technological advances.

▶ The setting of short-, medium-, and long-term goals is the spring which will set in motion any project, from the simplest to the most complex – e.g., in the short term, to do a certain number of workout sessions in a week; in the medium term, to change the level of exercise over the course of a month; in the long term, to lose several pounds over six months with the help of a balanced diet.

Learning how to breathe

"Learning how to breathe" sounds quite strange, because we believe that the act of breathing is so natural that it does not need to be relearned. It is something we do spontaneously from birth and is repeated a vast number of times over a lifetime. A newborn takes 60 to 70 breaths a minute; this number goes down to 26 at about age five, reaches 20 between ages ten and twenty, and settles at around 15 to 18 breaths per minute in adults. The vital capacity of an adult is about 4 quarts (4 liters) of air. In the paragraph on breathing (page 30) we saw how, based on gender and age, it undergoes variations, which influence its functionality. Rediscovering the correct way of breathing is of help not only for abdominal exercises, but also for restoration of your body's optimal fitness.

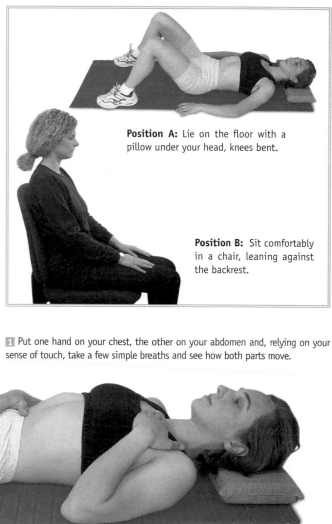

Position A: Lie on the floor with a pillow under your head, knees bent.

Position B: Sit comfortably in a chair, leaning against the backrest.

1 Put one hand on your chest, the other on your abdomen and, relying on your sense of touch, take a few simple breaths and see how both parts move.

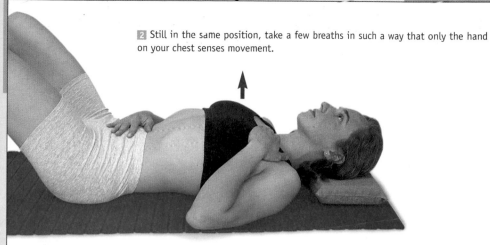

2 Still in the same position, take a few breaths in such a way that only the hand on your chest senses movement.

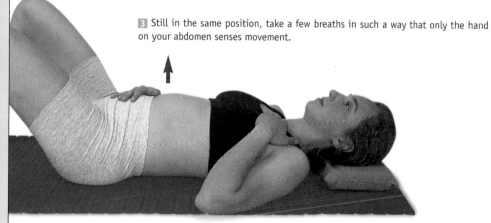

3 Still in the same position, take a few breaths in such a way that only the hand on your abdomen senses movement.

4 Still in that position, alternate Exercises #2 and #3, keeping your hands in place.

5 Still in the same position, try to exhale fully (push the air out your mouth) and to inhale deeply, doing both with the mouth open; as your belly pushes out and pulls in, you will realize that the abdominal muscles participate in this exercise.

Now that you're back in touch with your own breathing, let's try to use it correctly during the exercises.

Exercise cannot be done in a state of apnea (absence of breathing), which is why, while doing the exercises, at the exertion phase it is necessary to exhale, either by nose or mouth.

Normal breathing should be maintained during those exercises that call for holding a position without moving, to harmonize execution of the workout with the needs of your body.

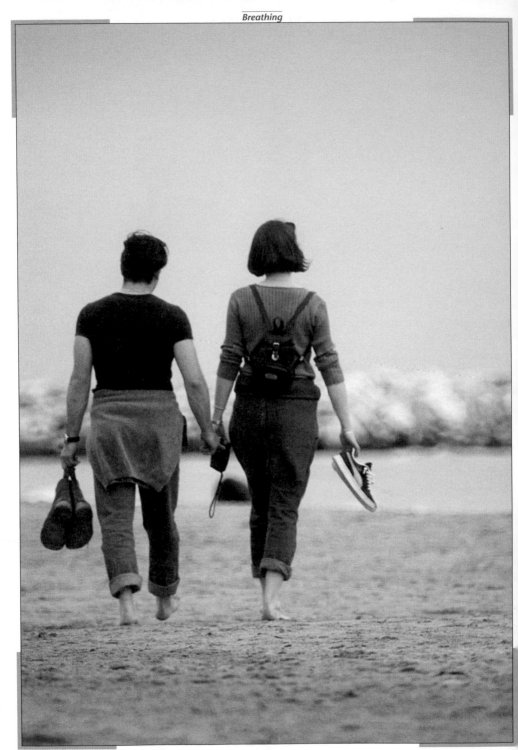

BEFORE STARTING

WORKOUT INSTRUCTIONS

A few simple suggestions will let you get good results from your workout program which, based on the instructions and on the initial test, will be better tailored to your needs and more easily introduced into your daily life. Those instructions are as follows:

▶ **Time**. Choose a time of day to exercise when you will be able to work calmly and in a relaxed fashion without being caught up in the daily preoccupations of phone calls, children, commitments, and studying. At the office, find time for a quiet break that will let you concentrate on yourself.

▶ **Clothing**. It's important to get rid of anything tight or binding which inhibits free breathing; wear comfortable clothes, which allow freedom of motion.

Take a break if you are at the office, finding a brief moment to reflect during the hectic pace of daily life. The space and location are not important as long as you feel good there and in harmony with your surroundings.

▶ **Frequency of workout**. Try to dedicate at least three times a week to working out, with each session at least 15 minutes long, because continuity of workout will allow you to maintain the effects of movement. There is no point in doing a prolonged workout only once a week. Too much time elapses before the next session, and you risk not maintaining the results achieved.

▶ **Listen to yourself**. Do all the exercises without pushing your physical exertion to the maximum; try instead to listen to the sensations of pleasure or pain your body is sending out. If you feel pain while doing the exercises, stop doing them or repeat them more carefully. Your workout must always start from your physical state, and it should be altered if your body's messages at that moment don't let you complete what you had planned.

▶ **Evaluation of the immediate effects**. If you have any doubts about your health and you feel overly tired even after a simple workout, or you have the sensation of labored breathing or pain in your muscles and joints, you must have a thorough medical checkup in order to avoid unpleasant surprises during your workout program.

CONSULTING THE BOOK

So that you will understand the workout, we explain the structure of the workout program. As you move on to practice, you will find the following useful:

▶ Three progressions of workout are given, differentiated by levels of difficulty of the exercises:
- **Level A**: easy exercises
- **Level B**: intermediate exercises
- **Level C**: complex exercises.

▶ There is a written description of each exercise, explaining the correct way of doing it, the most common mistakes, and the breathing pattern to follow.

▶ The layout of the text and numerous photographs let you visualize the exercises and how they are done. Once you've understood the exercise, the photographs alone will show you how to do it quickly with the best results.

▶ The workout repetitions and variations follow the suggestions in the paragraph on progressive overload (see page 19), but usually are listed in the exercise instructions also.

▶ To decide which exercises to do first, recall the things you did in the self-examination on pages 26 to 27.

▶ *If you had trouble doing the breathing exercises, were unable to hold the lowered sitting position for 20 seconds or to touch your elbows to your knees 10 times, start with the* **Level A** *exercises.*

▶ *If you were able to successfully perform the sitting exercises and to touch your knees with your elbows, start with the* **Level B** *exercises.*

▶ *The* **Level C** *exercises, which are the most difficult, are developed in stages over time as the fitness level is increased. They assume a knowledge of the movements and muscle control that you will get by completing at least one of the two preceding levels.*

STRUCTURE OF THE WORKOUTS

Taking your time into account, the workout you decide upon should be structured with the following sequence of exercises:
- Breathing exercises
- Exercises for the back (cervical, thoracic, lumbar, and overall mobility)
- Stretching exercises
- Warmup exercises
- Exercises for the abdominals.

▶ **The time** you devote to the session should be no less than 15 to 20 minutes, which will allow your body to benefit from the physiological changes that exercise generates.

The exercises suggested for the various stages are many, initially to allow for variation in the type of workout on different sectors of the abdominal muscles, but also to avoid the boredom which might set in doing the same motions over and over.

▶ It is important to determine the **number of exercises** to be done during the workout session.

For **breathing exercises**, follow the text instructions for each workout session.

For **back exercises**, it is important to do at least one exercise for each area involved (cervical, thoracic, lumbar, and overall).

For **stretching exercises**, follow the text instructions.

For **warmup exercises**, choose one sequence for each session.

For **abdominal exercises**, the subdivision into three levels, at least at the start, is as follows:

- **Level A exercises**: Starting with 6 repetitions of each exercise, add one repetition per week until reaching 10;
- **Level B exercises**: Starting with 6 repetitions of each exercise, add one repetition per week until reaching 10;
- **Level C exercises**: Starting with 6 repetitions of each exercise, add one repetition per week until reaching 10.

▶ **Passing from one level to the next** (e.g., from Level A to Level B) will involve starting with 6 repetitions, adding one repetition each week until reaching 10 and so on, as above.

Here's a practical example: If a person starts at Level A, he does 6 repetitions of each exercise and adds one repetition per week. After 4 weeks, he has reached 10 repetitions and then starts the Level B exercises with 6 repetitions until reaching 10, and so forth. When 10 repetitions of Level C are reached, he starts again at Level C, but this time with 10 repetitions, adding one every week until reaching 15; then he will start from 15 until reaching 20 repetitions. This effort involves a prolonged and constant commitment with the goal of creating a daily motor habit and increased muscle level stimulation. If you find yourself doing more than 25 repetitions, it could be that:

- The exercise is too easy
- It is being done in an incorrect manner.

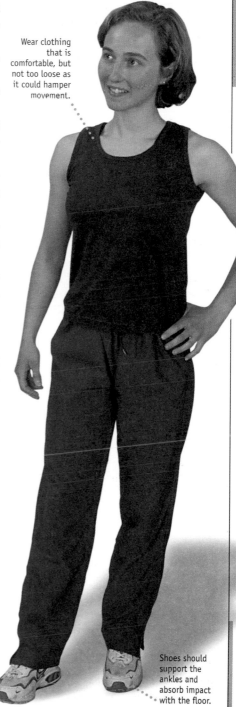

Wear clothing that is comfortable, but not too loose as it could hamper movement.

Shoes should support the ankles and absorb impact with the floor.

Breathing exercises

Two versions of these exercises are offered: one can be done at home, where you have the chance to stretch out and move about, and the other can be done at the office or other work situation, where space and clothing considerations may limit movement. Position A shows how the exercise should be done at home; Position B, at the office.

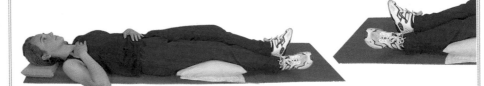

Position A: Lie flat with a cushion under your head and one under your knees, one hand on your chest and the other on your

Position B: Sit, leaning fully against the backrest, feet firmly on the floor, one hand on your chest and the other on your abdomen.

1 Inhale through your nose while lifting your chest, and try to feel the movement with your fingers. As you exhale, return to the starting position. Repeat 5 times.

2 Inhale as you distend your abdomen. As you exhale, return to the starting position. Repeat 5 times.

3 Breathe in through your nose, first expanding the abdomen, then continue inhaling until you feel the air enter your chest. At this point, hold your breath, then exhale. In this exercise, increase the breathing times, starting with 5 seconds breathing in, 3 seconds holding your breath, and 5 seconds breathing out. Repeat 5 times.

4 Now put your hands at the back of your neck. Breathe in, trying to spread your elbows as far apart as possible (those lying flat cannot go further than the floor; those sitting must be careful not to arch the back) and expand chest and abdomen. Exhale, returning to the starting position. Repeat 5 times.

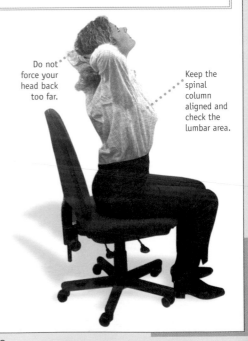

Do not force your head back too far.

Keep the spinal column aligned and check the lumbar area.

Back exercises

These exercises must be done very carefully before each session by everybody (the young, adults, beginners, or athletes) who plans to work out, but particularly by anybody who suffers from a so-called "bad back." All of these suggested exercises must be done carefully according to the instructions, never forcing any movement.

CERVICAL (NECK) MOBILITY

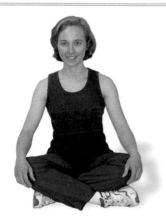

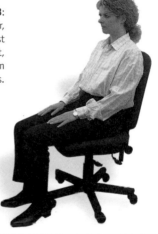

Position B: Sit in chair, back against backrest, hands on knees.

Position A: Sit with legs crossed, hands on knees.

1 Inhale; exhale, bending the head forward. Inhale again, returning to the starting position, keeping your head still. Repeat 6 times.

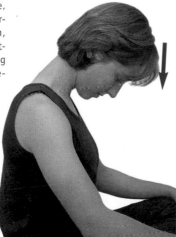

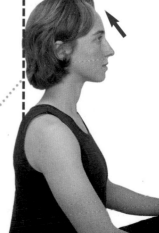

Do not bend your head back.

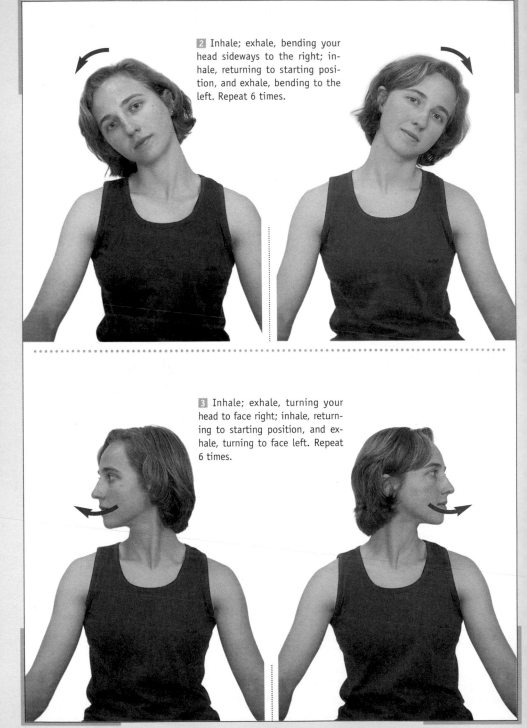

2 Inhale; exhale, bending your head sideways to the right; inhale, returning to starting position, and exhale, bending to the left. Repeat 6 times.

3 Inhale; exhale, turning your head to face right; inhale, returning to starting position, and exhale, turning to face left. Repeat 6 times.

THORACIC (CHEST) MOBILITY

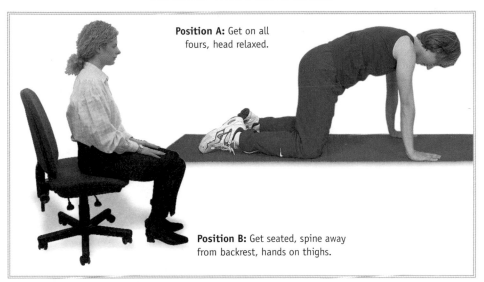

Position A: Get on all fours, head relaxed.

Position B: Get seated, spine away from backrest, hands on thighs.

1 Inhale; exhale and, pressing the back up, bend your head toward your arms. Inhale, letting the back drop back down and moving your head up. Repeat 6 times.

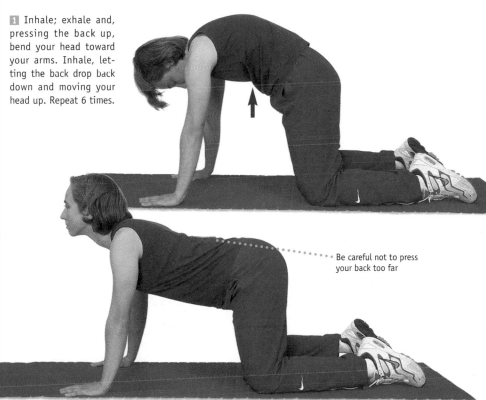

Be careful not to press your back too far

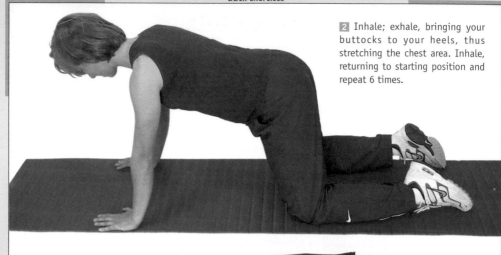

2 Inhale; exhale, bringing your buttocks to your heels, thus stretching the chest area. Inhale, returning to starting position and repeat 6 times.

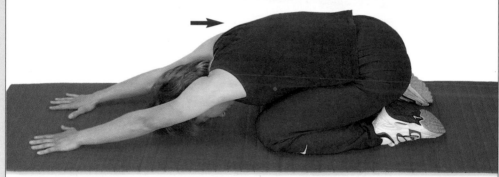

3 Inhale; exhale, bending your torso to the left, then inhale returning to the center and exhale, bending to the right. Repeat 6 times.

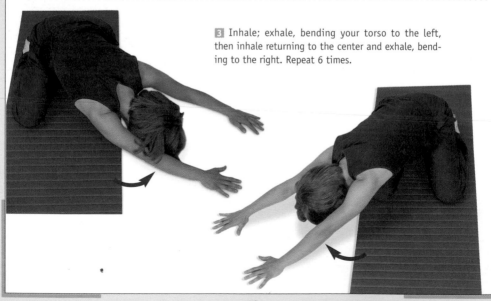

LUMBAR MOBILITY

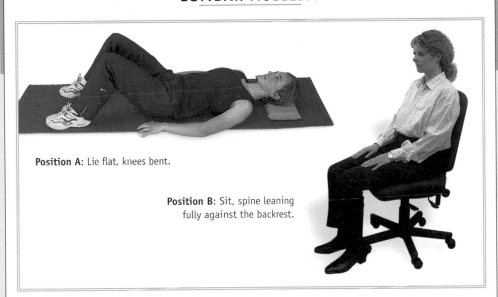

Position A: Lie flat, knees bent.

Position B: Sit, spine leaning fully against the backrest.

1 Inhale; exhale, bringing one bent leg to your chest, clasping it with both hands. Inhale, returning the leg and arms to the floor, and repeat with the other leg. Do this 10 times.

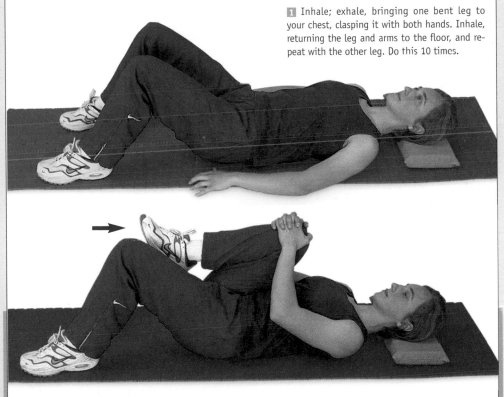

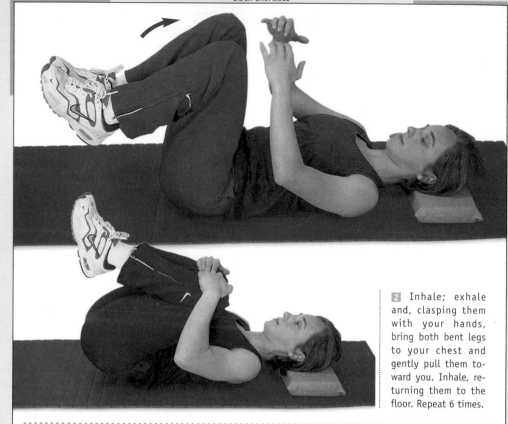

2 Inhale; exhale and, clasping them with your hands, bring both bent legs to your chest and gently pull them toward you. Inhale, returning them to the floor. Repeat 6 times.

3 Inhale; exhale, rotating your pelvis forward and up and trying to flatten the small of your back. Inhale and return to starting position. Do this 10 times.

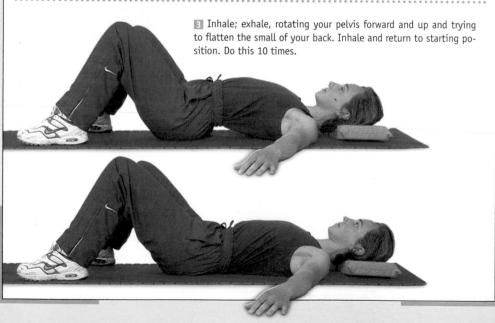

OVERALL MOBILITY

Position A: Lie flat, knees bent.

Position B: Stand with feet apart, arms at your sides.

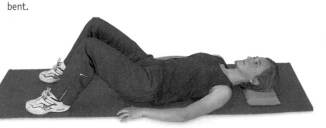

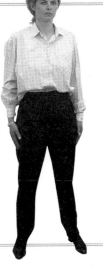

1 For Position A: Arms straight out to the sides. Inhale; exhale letting your relaxed, bent legs drop to the left and simultaneously turning your head to the right. Inhale and return to the starting position, then repeat on the other side. Do this 10 times.

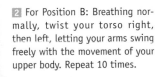

2 For Position B: Breathing normally, twist your torso right, then left, letting your arms swing freely with the movement of your upper body. Repeat 10 times.

Stretching exercises

This category of exercises also merits a few words, given its importance in any workout program. Stretching exercises permit us to relax our contracted, tense muscles, to check their hardness and, not least of all, to find the proper breathing rhythm, which is so important.

To do these exercises better, bear in mind the following:

- Never force stretching to the point of pain;
- Never "bounce" (an absolutely incorrect movement, particularly from a physiological point of view) with the idea you'll get better results;
- Carefully follow the signals your muscles are sending out and never try to ignore them.

EXERCISE #1

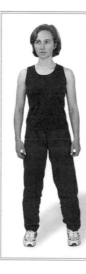

Position A:
Stand with feet apart, knees slightly bent.

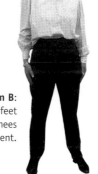

Position B:
Stand with feet apart, knees slightly bent.

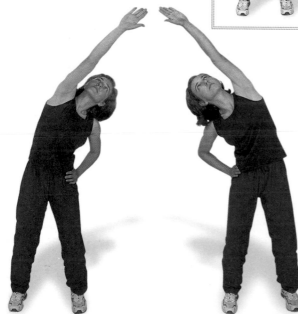

1 Inhale; exhale, stretching your right arm up, left hand on left hip, and bending left from the waist. Inhale, returning to starting position; then exhale while repeating to the other side. Do this 10 times.

46

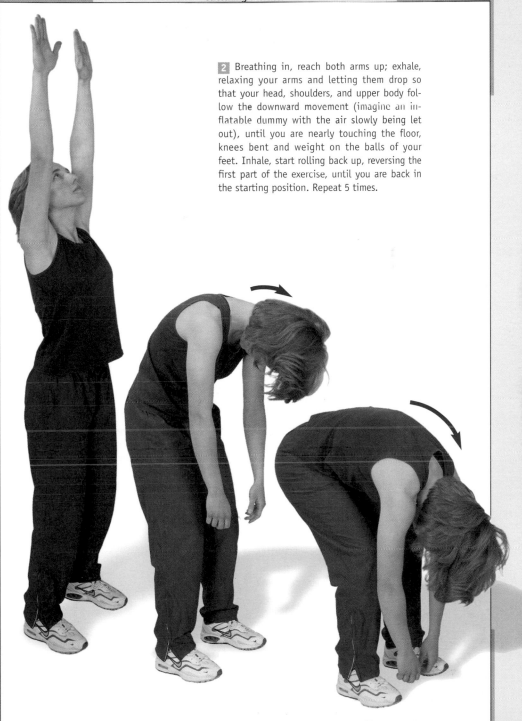

2 Breathing in, reach both arms up; exhale, relaxing your arms and letting them drop so that your head, shoulders, and upper body follow the downward movement (imagine an inflatable dummy with the air slowly being let out), until you are nearly touching the floor, knees bent and weight on the balls of your feet. Inhale, start rolling back up, reversing the first part of the exercise, until you are back in the starting position. Repeat 5 times.

EXERCISE #2

Position A: Sit with knees bent, soles of feet together, hands on your toes.

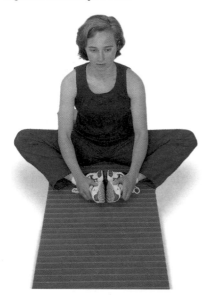

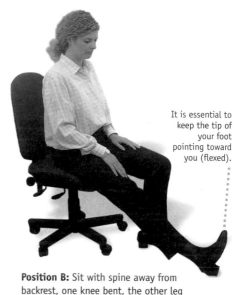

It is essential to keep the tip of your foot pointing toward you (flexed).

Position B: Sit with spine away from backrest, one knee bent, the other leg extended toward the floor.

1 For Position A: Inhale; exhale, slowly stretching your right leg out straight on the floor, your hand still on your foot, letting your torso follow the movement. Inhale, return to the starting position, then repeat with the left leg. Repeat 5 times per leg.

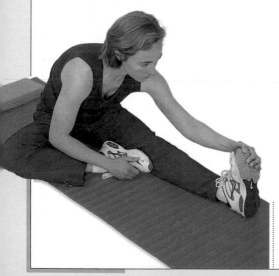

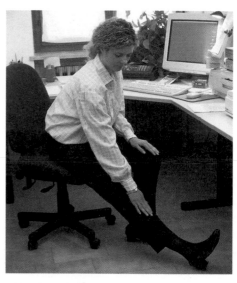

2 For Position B: Inhale; exhale, bending your upper body forward and reaching toward your feet. Inhale, returning to starting position; repeat with the other leg. Repeat 5 times per leg.

EXERCISE #3

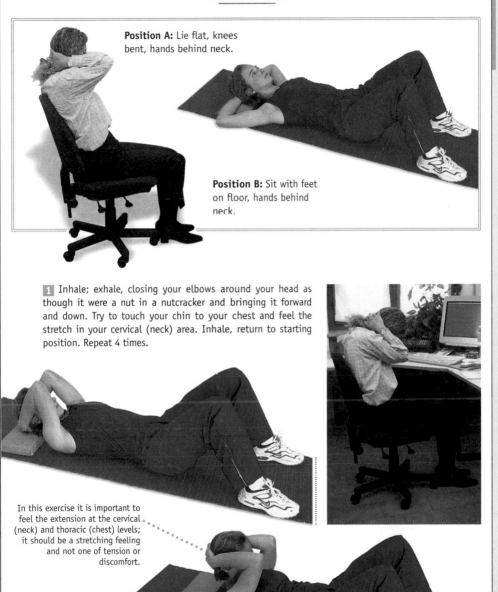

Position A: Lie flat, knees bent, hands behind neck.

Position B: Sit with feet on floor, hands behind neck.

1 Inhale; exhale, closing your elbows around your head as though it were a nut in a nutcracker and bringing it forward and down. Try to touch your chin to your chest and feel the stretch in your cervical (neck) area. Inhale, return to starting position. Repeat 4 times.

In this exercise it is important to feel the extension at the cervical (neck) and thoracic (chest) levels; it should be a stretching feeling and not one of tension or discomfort.

Warmup exercises

To begin working your muscles in a positive physiological way, it is important to warm up sufficiently, so that the body can easily withstand the muscle toning program it is about to undertake. The warmup exercises you choose should be rhythmic and continuous, thus allowing you to stimulate the cardiovascular system in a progressive and steady manner. You might take a walk or jog in place, but this runs the risk of making the warmup boring and not very stimulating. An alternative would be to warm up to some of your favorite music; or, if that's not possible, hum a pleasant rhythm to yourself; in any case, an enjoyable background will kill the boredom that is lying in wait while you exercise. Be careful not to put a strain on your heart. In fact, if you start an intense workout from a resting state, you run the risk that the myocardial circulatory system, which feeds the heart, might not supply enough blood (a condition known as cardioischemia), with consequences that can be easily overcome by somebody in shape, but that could create serious problems for a beginner, particularly one who has heart disease. The warmup will consist of progressing from light activity (pulse of 90 to 100 beats per minute) to moderate activity (120 beats per minute) for a period that will gradually increase from 5 to 10 minutes.

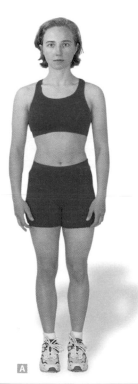

EXERCISE #1

From the starting position, which you can see in Photograph A, hop once to the left (B), take two hops to the right (C), one hop backward (D), and one forward (E), returning to the starting position.

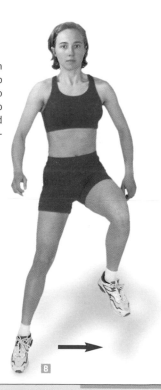

A

B

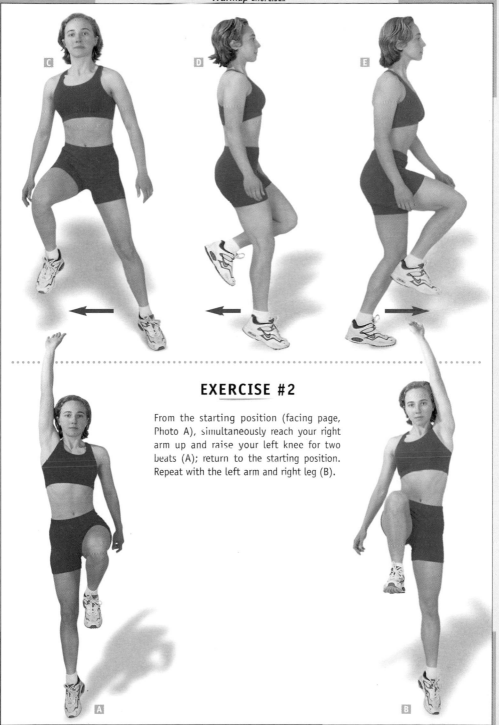

EXERCISE #2

From the starting position (facing page, Photo A), simultaneously reach your right arm up and raise your left knee for two beats (A); return to the starting position. Repeat with the left arm and right leg (B).

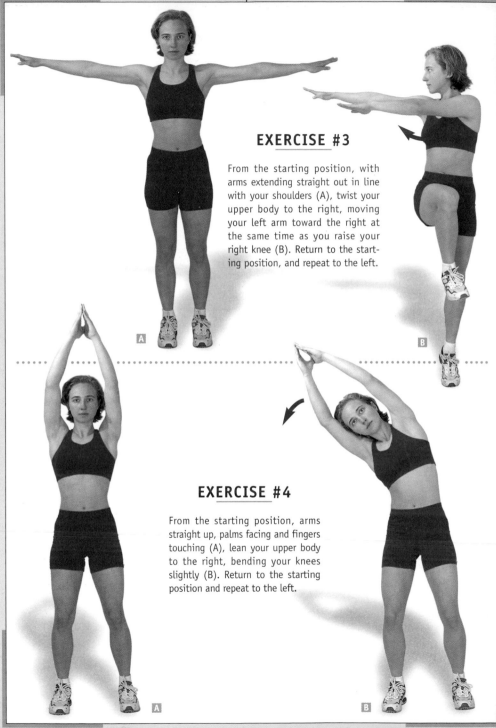

EXERCISE #3

From the starting position, with arms extending straight out in line with your shoulders (A), twist your upper body to the right, moving your left arm toward the right at the same time as you raise your right knee (B). Return to the starting position, and repeat to the left.

EXERCISE #4

From the starting position, arms straight up, palms facing and fingers touching (A), lean your upper body to the right, bending your knees slightly (B). Return to the starting position and repeat to the left.

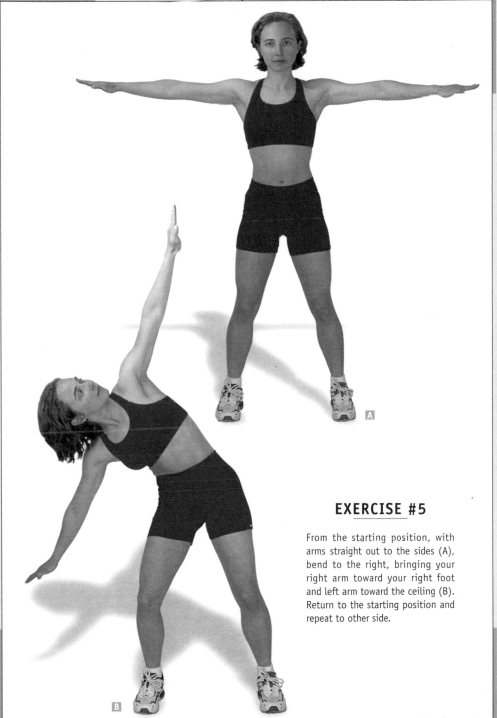

EXERCISE #5

From the starting position, with arms straight out to the sides (A), bend to the right, bringing your right arm toward your right foot and left arm toward the ceiling (B). Return to the starting position and repeat to other side.

53

EXERCISES FOR THE ABDOMINALS

There are a great number of books about exercises for abdominal muscles, and our imaginations might suggest ever more complicated and spectacular exercises, which might yield astonishing results. (We all remember the films about a boxer who went through training exercises that were unbelievable and undoable by ordinary people.)

Many books are written by athletic trainers, by athletes wanting to put their personal experiences in writing, or by physical therapists who work directly in restoring functionality to individuals who have suffered accidents or trauma.

The majority of people, probably including yourself, do not fall into the category of athlete or someone who wants to become a trainer. You probably have not suffered any trauma, nor do you have to recover from a physical injury. So why bore you with instructions and suggestions that

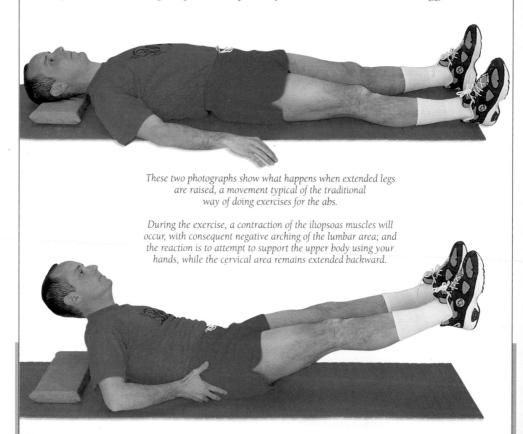

These two photographs show what happens when extended legs are raised, a movement typical of the traditional way of doing exercises for the abs.

During the exercise, a contraction of the iliopsoas muscles will occur, with consequent negative arching of the lumbar area; and the reaction is to attempt to support the upper body using your hands, while the cervical area remains extended backward.

do not concern you directly? For this reason, we start with basic exercises, from which all the others will be developed, aimed at a more diverse audience – from the mere mortal with a little paunch to the athlete who is ready for the Olympics.

rectly (see photos on page 54). If you ask someone who is out of shape to sit up from a prone position, he will have problems doing the exercise, because the intensity of the motion is not gradual. Our basic exercise consists of lying prone from a

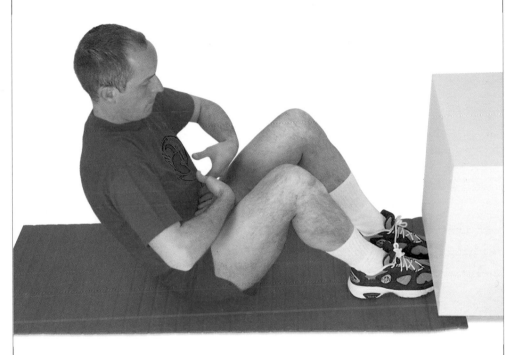

▶ Abdominal muscles are muscles with a tendency to contract isometrically (with no change in length) and not isotonical-ly (with variation in length) as the majority of the muscles of the body do. Each time you rise from a sitting or prone position (lying down), you tend to involve the iliopsoas muscles, creating excessive tension in the lower back, without the abdominal muscles being involved. This happens frequently when the standard exercise for toning abdominal muscles is not done cor-

Doing the exercise by moving down from a sitting position allows you to control the movement of the abdominal muscles and at the same time feel them working.

sitting position, an exercise which offers a dual advantage. First, it has gradual intensity, compared to sitting up from a prone position, because as you lower yourself, you can stop at the point at which you run into difficulty, making the exercise personalized. Second, you can identify the work of your abdominal muscles, especially in the first phase, by touching your muscles as they are stimulated by movement. The muscles react to the exercise, sending a signal (photo above).

▶ Sit with knees bent, feet immobilized under a piece of furniture, head inclined forward, and hands on stomach in such a way that the fingers can feel the muscles.

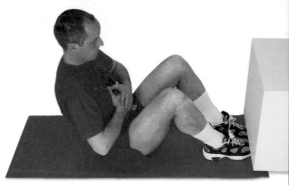

Hands on stomach let you feel the abdominal muscles.

▶ Breathing normally, without holding your breath, slowly lean back until you have the feeling of exerting moderate effort, or continue going downwards until you get this feeling. If the effort is excessive, lie back down on the floor and, using your hands, return to a sitting position and repeat the exercise. At this point the toning process starts. This position should be held for 15 to 20 seconds, until your muscles tend to tremble. With training, this hold time will get longer and longer, giving you an additional sign of your improved physical fitness.

When you can hold this position for 20 seconds without getting muscle tremors, you will be able to lie back until you are almost touching the floor.

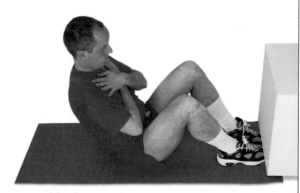

With hands on your chest, progressive overload increases.

▶ At this point it is possible to increase the progressive overload by involving your arms. Until now the upper limbs were used only to let your hands feel the muscle contractions; now they will change position, as shown at right.

▶ When you have reached the goal and changed position, start over again, holding the position for 15 seconds, so that each time the position will be more difficult to hold.

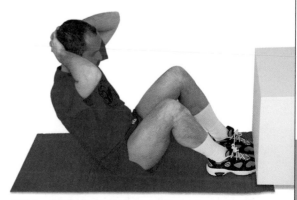

With hands behind your head, progressive overload is significant, so be careful not to do this exercise incorrectly.

Level A exercises

EXERCISE #1

Flat on back, knees bent, arms relaxed, feet on the floor. Inhale; exhale, contracting the abdominal muscles, flattening out the lumbar arch, and slightly lifting the pubic area. Hold this position. Inhale, relax, and repeat.

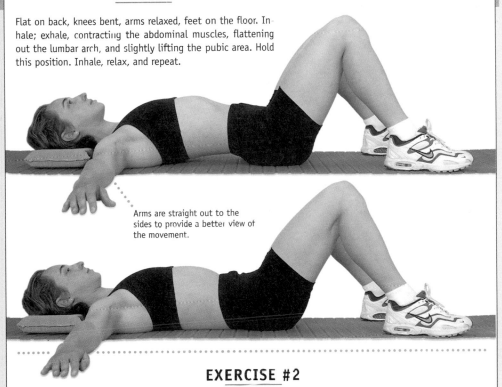

Arms are straight out to the sides to provide a better view of the movement.

EXERCISE #2

Feet immobilized under a piece of furniture (bed, sofa, desk), knees bent, thighs near calves, hands on stomach, and head leaning forward. Inhale; as you exhale, slowly lean back (without arching your back), holding for 10 to 15 seconds to the point where you feel a slight strain. When fatigue or muscle tremors are felt, inhale, sit back up, and repeat.

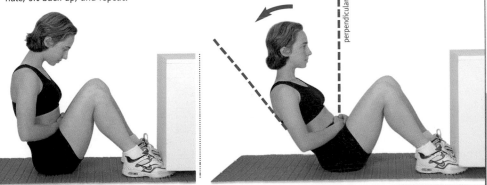

perpendicular

EXERCISE #3

Lie flat, knees bent, soles of feet on floor, hands behind head, elbows parallel. Inhale; exhale and, using your arms to help, raise head and shoulders from the floor without arching back. Relax as you inhale, and repeat.

EXERCISE #4

Lie flat, hands behind head, elbows open, left knee bent, left foot on floor, right leg resting on left knee. Inhale; exhale and, using your right elbow for leverage, lift head and chest, bringing the left elbow toward the right knee. Inhale, lying back down. Repeat on the other side.

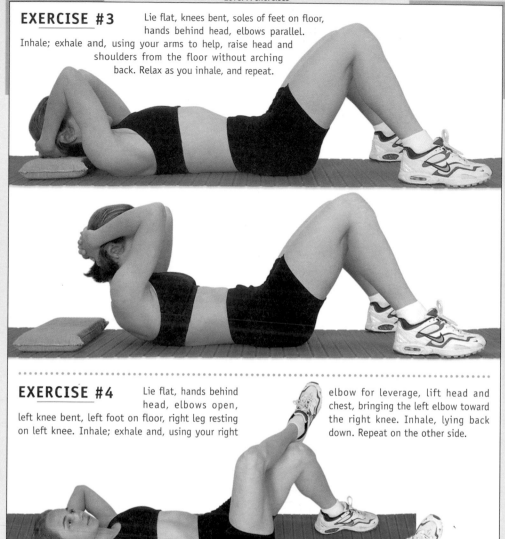

EXERCISE #5

Lie flat, knees bent, soles of feet on floor, arms flat above your head. Inhale and exhale, inflating (when inhaling) and deflating (when exhaling) the abdomen and contracting the abs as you exhale.

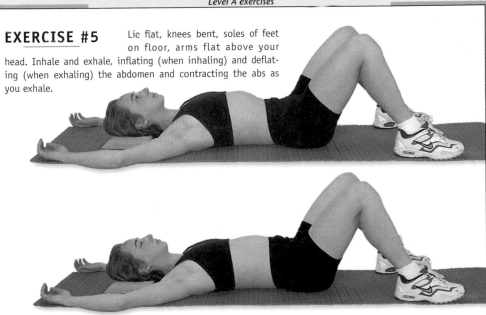

EXERCISE #6

Lie flat, knees bent, soles of feet on floor, arms at sides, palms touching floor. Inhale; exhale, bringing bent knees toward head and trying to raise buttocks off the floor. Inhale, returning to the floor, and repeat.

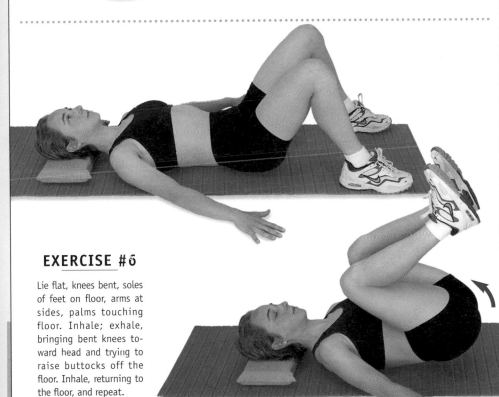

EXERCISE #7

Lie on your back, knees bent, lower legs resting on chair seat or stool, hands holding the backs of thighs.

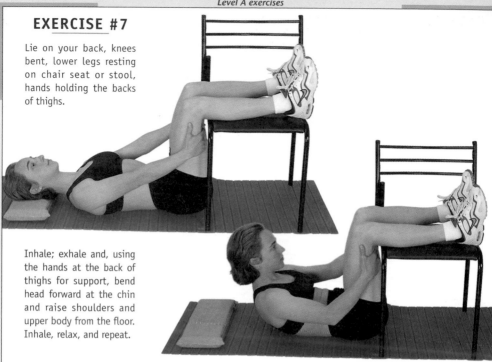

Inhale; exhale and, using the hands at the back of thighs for support, bend head forward at the chin and raise shoulders and upper body from the floor. Inhale, relax, and repeat.

EXERCISE #8

Lie on right side, head resting on right hand, right elbow on the floor, right knee bent, right leg in front of body, left leg extended to floor. Inhale; exhale, lifting left leg in line with upper body. Inhale, relax, and repeat. Do 6 repetitions; then change to left side.

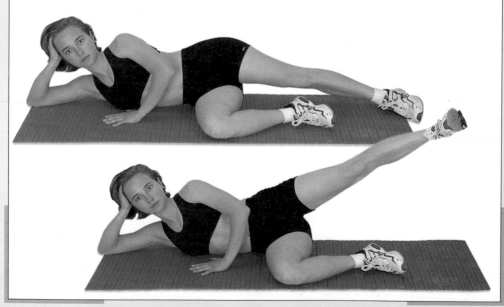

EXERCISE #9

Lie on back, hands behind head, knees bent, feet on floor. Inhale; exhale, raising bent right knee and upper body, supporting head with arms, and bring all toward the midline. Inhale, relax, and repeat with the other leg.

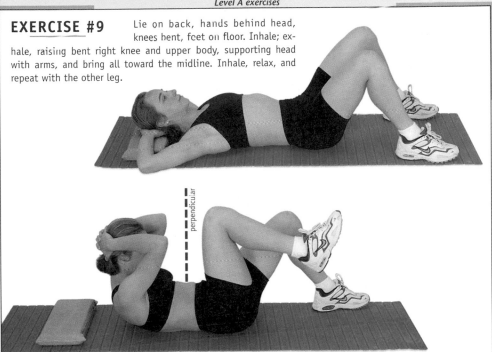

perpendicular

EXERCISE #10

Kneeling on the floor, sit back on your heels, arms stretched forward, with back straight. Inhale; exhale, lifting buttocks and shifting them to the right until you are sitting on the floor, then twist arms to the left. Inhale, returning to center position sitting on heels, and exhale, repeating exercise to the left. Repeat 6 times.

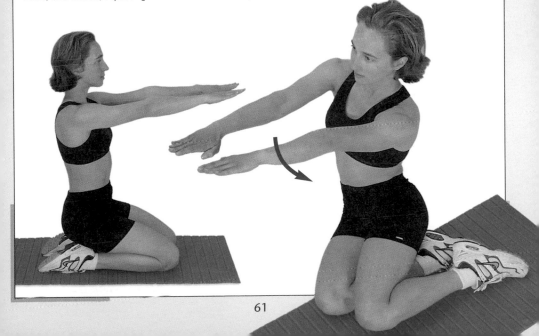

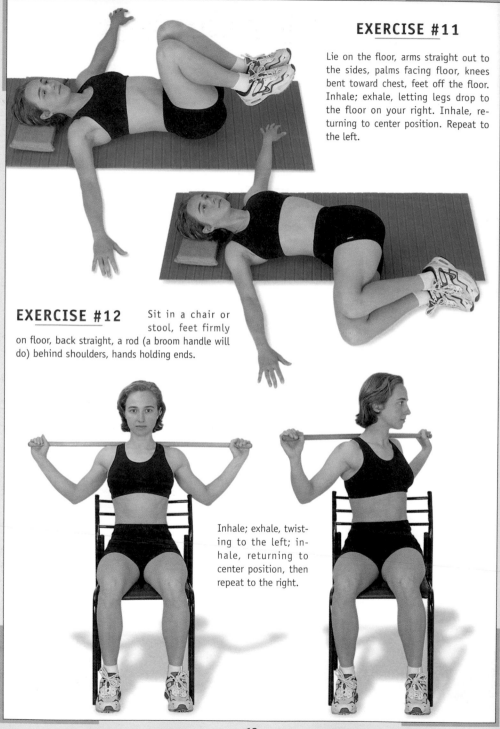

EXERCISE #11

Lie on the floor, arms straight out to the sides, palms facing floor, knees bent toward chest, feet off the floor. Inhale; exhale, letting legs drop to the floor on your right. Inhale, returning to center position. Repeat to the left.

EXERCISE #12

Sit in a chair or stool, feet firmly on floor, back straight, a rod (a broom handle will do) behind shoulders, hands holding ends.

Inhale; exhale, twisting to the left; inhale, returning to center position, then repeat to the right.

Level B exercises

EXERCISE #1

Stand with back against a wall, knees slightly bent, arms at sides. Inhale; exhale, flattening the small of your back against the wall and raising the pelvis slightly. Hold this position as you exhale. Inhale, relax, and repeat.

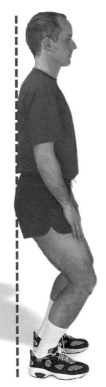
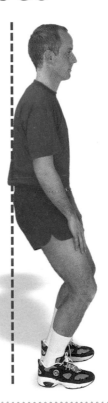

EXERCISE #2

Sit on floor, feet immobilized under a piece of furniture, knees bent, calves and thighs almost touching, hands on chest and head bent forward. Inhale; exhale, slowly leaning back (without arching spine), stopping for 10 to 15 seconds at the point where you feel a slight strain. When overexertion and muscle tremors set in, inhale, sit back up, and repeat.

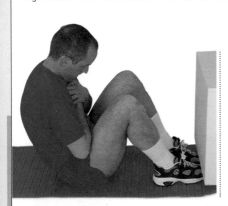
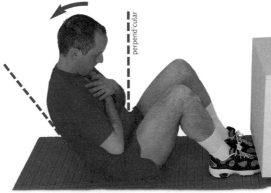

EXERCISE #3

Lie on the floor, knees bent, feet on floor, arms by sides. Inhale; exhale, raising head, shoulders, and arms, and try to touch thighs. Inhale, lying back down, and repeat.

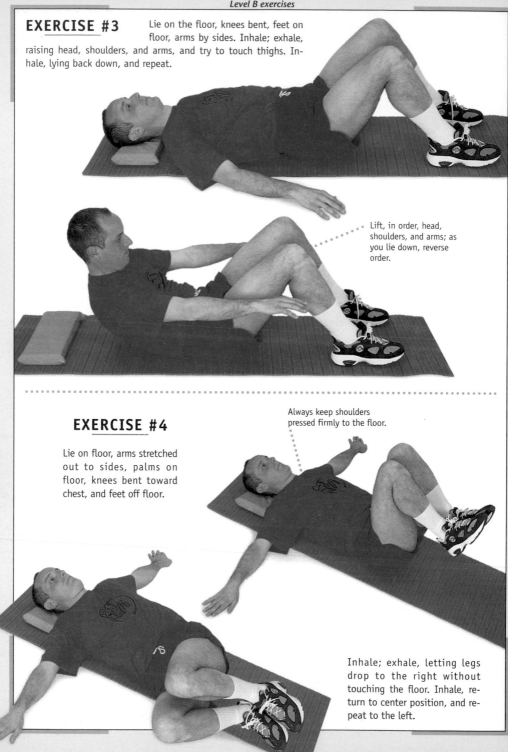

Lift, in order, head, shoulders, and arms; as you lie down, reverse order.

EXERCISE #4

Lie on floor, arms stretched out to sides, palms on floor, knees bent toward chest, and feet off floor.

Always keep shoulders pressed firmly to the floor.

Inhale; exhale, letting legs drop to the right without touching the floor. Inhale, return to center position, and repeat to the left.

EXERCISE #5

Lie on the floor, hands behind head, knees bent, feet on the floor. Inhale and exhale very rapidly from your diaphragm, inflating and deflating your belly 6 times.

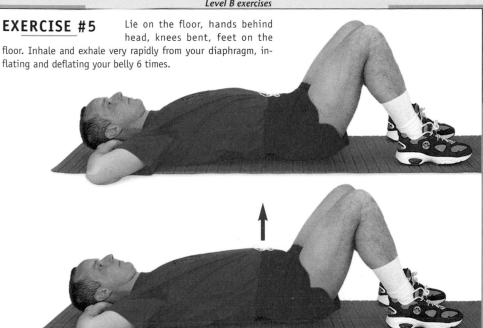

EXERCISE #6

Lie on the floor, knees bent toward chest, feet off the ground, weight on forearms. Breathing normally, alternately extend legs straight ahead (as for bicycle-pedaling) 6 times.

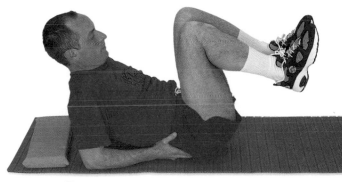

To avoid arching the lumbar area, do not lower legs too far.

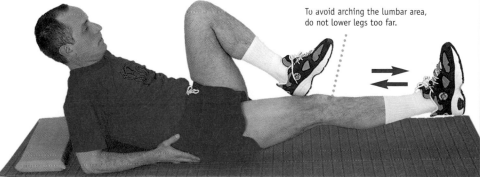

65

EXERCISE #7

Lie on back, knees bent, lower legs resting on chair, arms stretched upward. Inhale; exhale, bringing arms upward and forward and chest toward knees. Inhale, lie back down, and repeat.

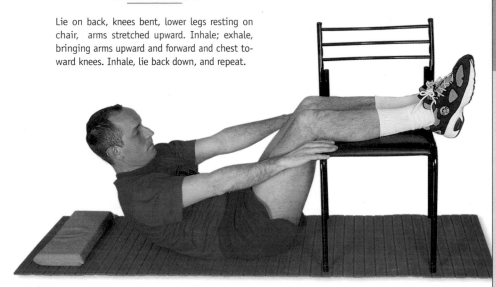

EXERCISE #8

Lie on your right side, head resting in right hand, right elbow on the floor, both legs extended beneath you. Inhale; exhale, lifting both legs and keeping them in line with torso. Inhale, relax, and repeat.

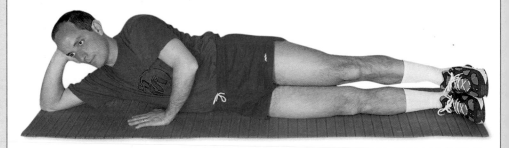

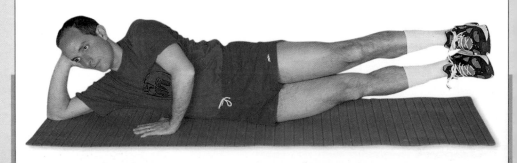

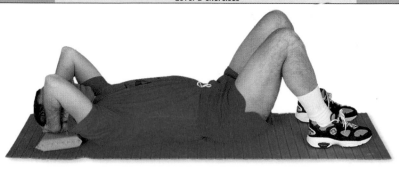

EXERCISE #9

Lie on back, hands behind head, feet on the floor. Inhale; exhale, lifting both bent knees and upper body and bringing them together (without going beyond perpendicular). Inhale, relax, and repeat.

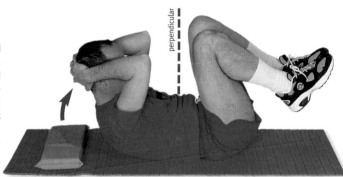

perpendicular

EXERCISE #10

Kneel on floor (sitting back on heels), arms crossed in front of chest, back straight. Inhale; exhale, moving buttocks to the right at the same time you move arms to the left. Inhale, return to starting position, and exhale, sitting over to the left. Repeat 6 times.

EXERCISE #11

Lie on back, arms straight out at sides, palms facing floor, right leg extended upward, left knee bent, foot off floor. Inhale; exhale, letting the right leg drop to the side without touching floor. Inhale, return to center position, and change sides. Repeat 6 times.

EXERCISE #12

Sit on a chair, feet firmly on floor, back straight, holding a stick behind shoulders.

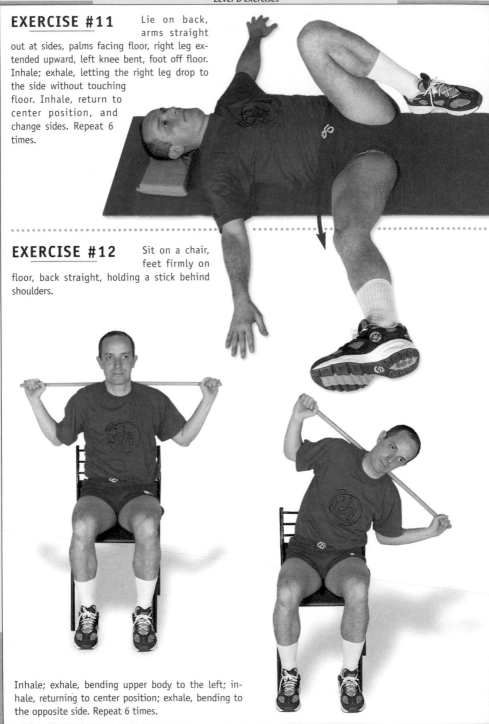

Inhale; exhale, bending upper body to the left; inhale, returning to center position; exhale, bending to the opposite side. Repeat 6 times.

Level C exercises

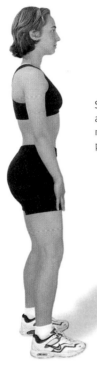

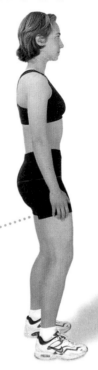

EXERCISE #1

Stand, legs slightly apart, knees bent, lumbar area flat as you exhale, contracting abdominal muscles and buttocks. Inhale, bringing the pelvis back to starting position.

See Exercise #1 of Level B. You need to assume and maintain the correct position, as though you were leaning against a wall.

EXERCISE #2

Sit on the floor, feet immobilized under a piece of furniture, hands behind head, fingers laced, head bent forward, and thighs near calves. Inhale; exhale, slowly lying back down (without arching back), stopping for 10 to 15 seconds at the point where you feel moderate strain. When fatigue or tremors set in, stop and sit up.

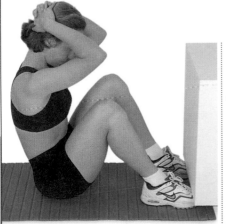

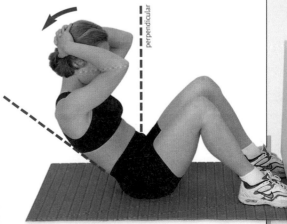

perpendicular

EXERCISE #3

Lie on the floor, right knee bent, left leg extended on the floor, and arms at sides. Inhale; exhale, simultaneously raising upper body and left leg, trying to touch your left toe with your right hand. Inhale, lie back on floor, and repeat exercise on the other side.

Always keep one knee bent for correct performance of this exercise.

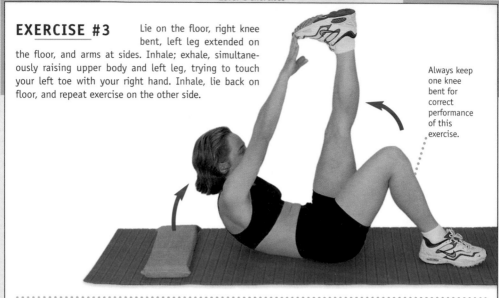

EXERCISE #4

Lie on back, torso pressed to floor, legs spread forward and raised up, knees slightly bent. Inhale; exhale, raising upper body and bringing hands toward right foot. Inhale, lying back down, and repeat exercise on the other side.

During this exercise, your legs should never move.

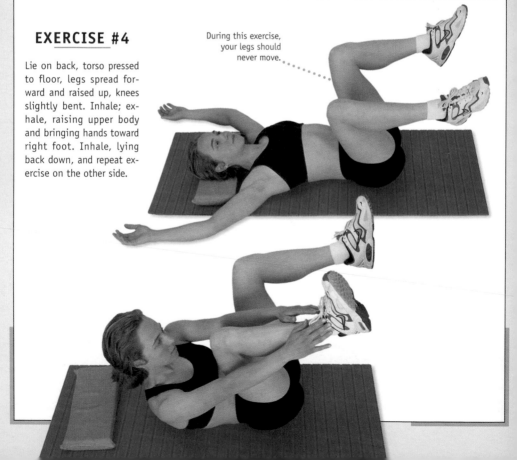

EXERCISE #5

Lie on floor, pull knees to your chest with the help of laced fingers. Inhale and exhale from the abdomen very rapidly while holding this position, 6 times.

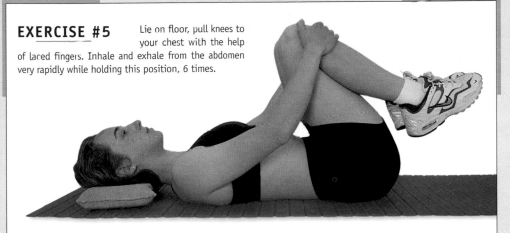

EXERCISE #6

Sit on the floor, knees bent toward chest, feet off the floor, weight on forearms. Inhale; exhale and, without arching the lumbar area, extend legs forward and up. Inhale, return to starting position, and repeat.

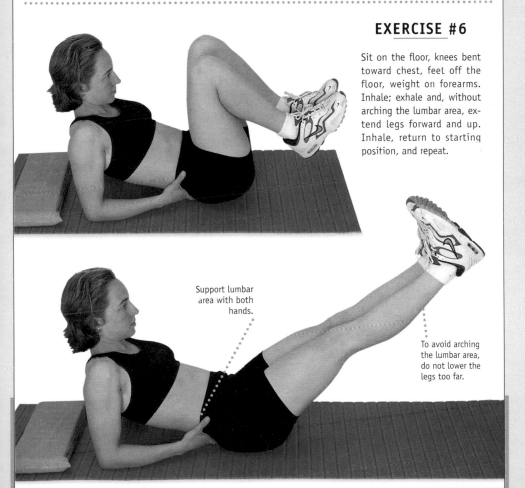

Support lumbar area with both hands.

To avoid arching the lumbar area, do not lower the legs too far.

EXERCISE #7

Lie on back, knees bent, lower legs resting on chair, hands behind head, elbows together.

Inhale; exhale, raising head, shoulders, and chest, and try to bring elbows to knees. Inhale, lying back down.

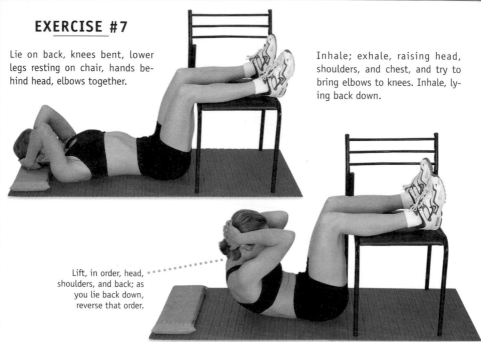

Lift, in order, head, shoulders, and back; as you lie back down, reverse that order.

EXERCISE #8

Lie on side, feet immobilized under a piece of furniture, knees slightly bent, arms extended over head, palms together.

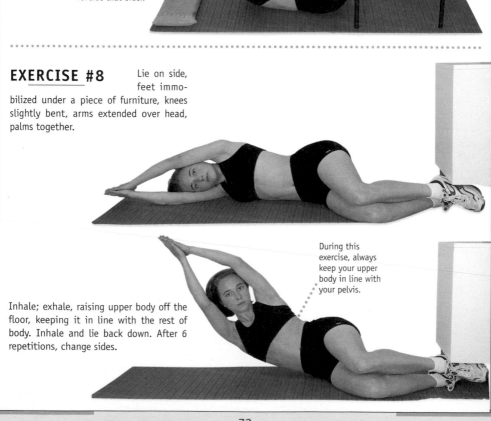

During this exercise, always keep your upper body in line with your pelvis.

Inhale; exhale, raising upper body off the floor, keeping it in line with the rest of body. Inhale and lie back down. After 6 repetitions, change sides.

EXERCISE #9

Lie on the floor, arms over head, left knee bent and right leg extended upward.

Keep the extended leg from moving during this exercise.

Inhale; exhale, raising arms, head, shoulders, and chest and trying to touch your outstretched foot. Inhale, lying back down; then repeat with the other leg.

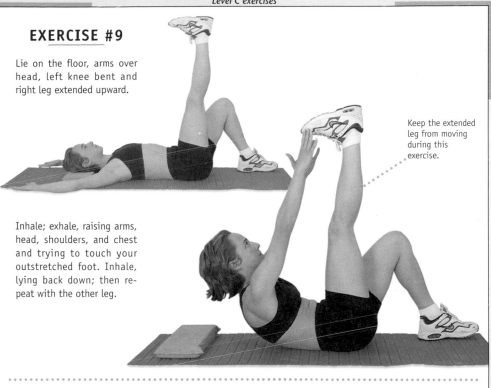

EXERCISE #10

Sit balanced on your buttocks, knees bent, arms extended in front. Inhale; exhale, twisting arms to the right and legs to the left. Inhale, return to center position, and repeat on other side.

Do not arch the lumbar area.

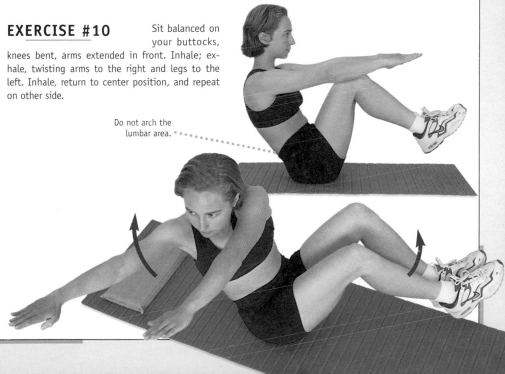

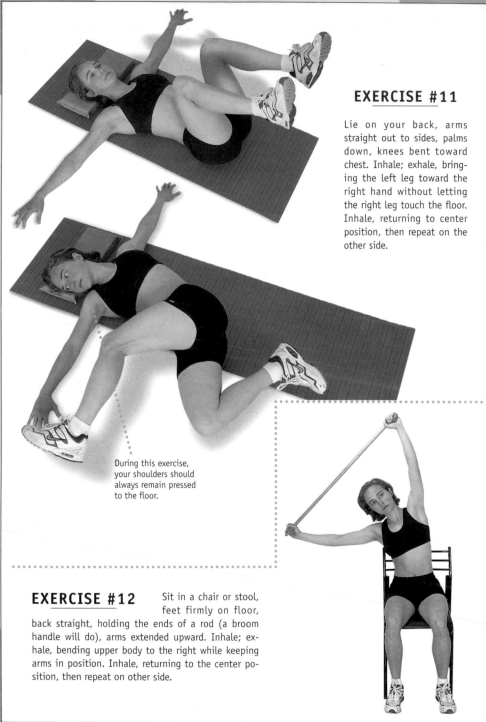

EXERCISE #11

Lie on your back, arms straight out to sides, palms down, knees bent toward chest. Inhale; exhale, bringing the left leg toward the right hand without letting the right leg touch the floor. Inhale, returning to center position, then repeat on the other side.

During this exercise, your shoulders should always remain pressed to the floor.

EXERCISE #12

Sit in a chair or stool, feet firmly on floor, back straight, holding the ends of a rod (a broom handle will do), arms extended upward. Inhale; exhale, bending upper body to the right while keeping arms in position. Inhale, returning to the center position, then repeat on other side.

Exercises at the office

When there is no time to go to the gym, and it's almost impossible to find space at home to work out, the office can become a place to do some exercises. Particularly if you work at a computer, it is important that you do the stretching exercises on pages 46 to 49. What about clothing? With these exercises, you can even work out wearing office clothes.

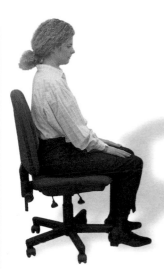

EXERCISE #1

Sit, back leaning against backrest, hands on thighs, feet firmly on floor. Inhale; exhale, forcibly contracting your abdominal musculature, sucking in your abdomen. Inhale and relax. Repeat 10 times.

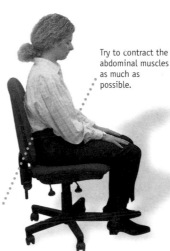

Try to contract the abdominal muscles as much as possible.

While exhaling, make sure the lumbar area is pressed firmly against the backrest.

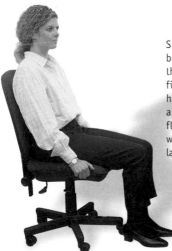

EXERCISE #2

Sit, back leaning against backrest, hands gripping the sides of the chair, feet firmly on the floor. Inhale; exhale, raising knees and lifting feet off the floor, bringing legs toward chest. Inhale and relax. Repeat 6 times.

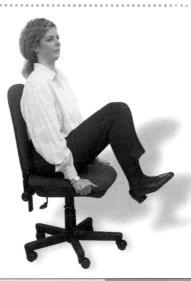

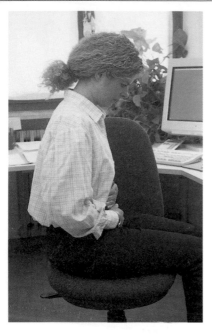

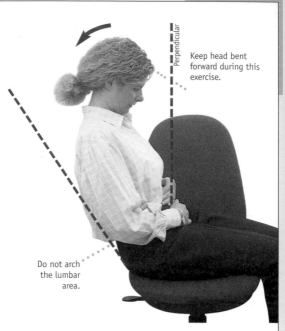

Perpendicular

Keep head bent forward during this exercise.

Do not arch the lumbar area.

EXERCISE #3

Sit sideways in the chair without using the backrest, feet firmly on the floor, hands on stomach and head bent forward. Inhale, exhale, leaning the upper body backwards at a 15- to 20-degree angle, and feel your muscles contract, without arching your back. Hold the position for 5 seconds and then sit up, breathing in. Repeat 6 times.

EXERCISE #4

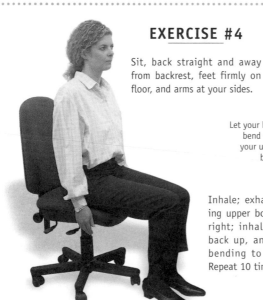

Sit, back straight and away from backrest, feet firmly on floor, and arms at your sides.

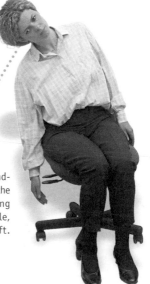

Let your head bend with your upper body.

Inhale; exhale, bending upper body to the right; inhale, sitting back up, and exhale, bending to the left. Repeat 10 times.

EXERCISE #5

Sit, back away from backrest, feet firmly on the floor, hands on hips. Inhale; exhale, twisting your upper body to the right; inhale, return to the center position, and exhale, twisting to the left. Repeat 10 times.

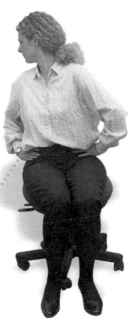

Let your head follow the movement of your upper body.

EXERCISE #6

Sit, back away from backrest, feet on the floor, hands gripping the sides of the chair. Inhale; exhale, simultaneously lifting feet, knees, and buttocks up, contracting abdominal muscles. Inhale and relax. Repeat 6 times.

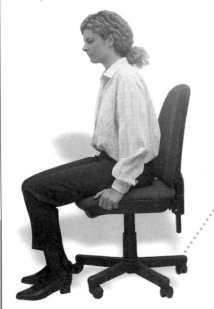

Do not hold your breath!

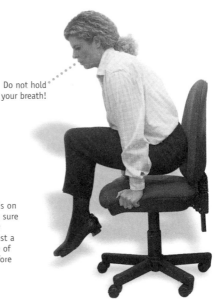

If the chair is on rollers, make sure it is securely braced against a wall or piece of furniture before doing this exercise.

PREGNANCY PROGRAM

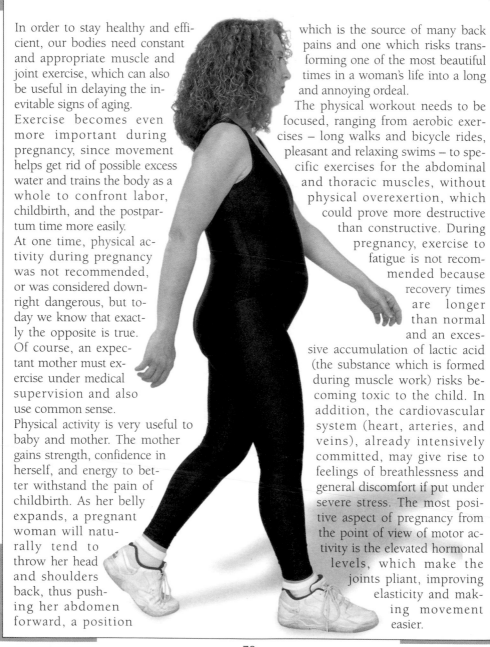

In order to stay healthy and efficient, our bodies need constant and appropriate muscle and joint exercise, which can also be useful in delaying the inevitable signs of aging. Exercise becomes even more important during pregnancy, since movement helps get rid of possible excess water and trains the body as a whole to confront labor, childbirth, and the postpartum time more easily.

At one time, physical activity during pregnancy was not recommended, or was considered downright dangerous, but today we know that exactly the opposite is true. Of course, an expectant mother must exercise under medical supervision and also use common sense.

Physical activity is very useful to baby and mother. The mother gains strength, confidence in herself, and energy to better withstand the pain of childbirth. As her belly expands, a pregnant woman will naturally tend to throw her head and shoulders back, thus pushing her abdomen forward, a position which is the source of many back pains and one which risks transforming one of the most beautiful times in a woman's life into a long and annoying ordeal.

The physical workout needs to be focused, ranging from aerobic exercises – long walks and bicycle rides, pleasant and relaxing swims – to specific exercises for the abdominal and thoracic muscles, without physical overexertion, which could prove more destructive than constructive. During pregnancy, exercise to fatigue is not recommended because recovery times are longer than normal and an excessive accumulation of lactic acid (the substance which is formed during muscle work) risks becoming toxic to the child. In addition, the cardiovascular system (heart, arteries, and veins), already intensively committed, may give rise to feelings of breathlessness and general discomfort if put under severe stress. The most positive aspect of pregnancy from the point of view of motor activity is the elevated hormonal levels, which make the joints pliant, improving elasticity and making movement easier.

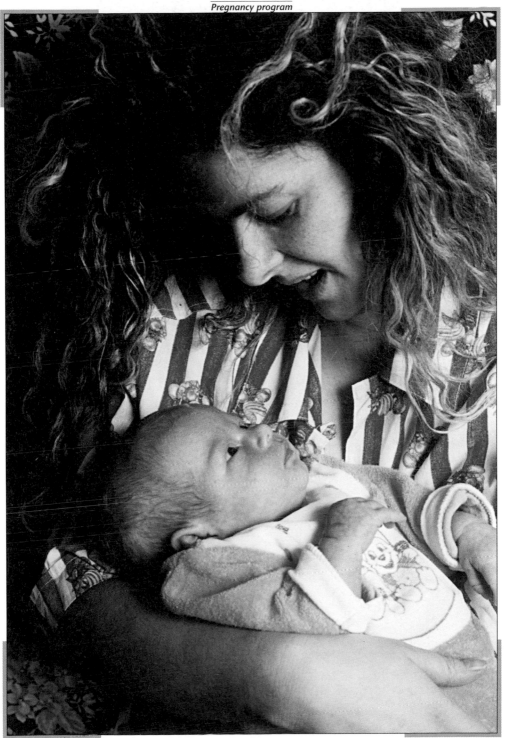

HOW TO MOVE

Here are a few instructions on the correct way to perform activities such as swimming and walking.

▶ While walking, pay attention to your body position, maintaining posture with back straight, shoulders back and relaxed, and arms loose at your sides so they can follow your movements.

▶ Wear comfortable shoes with good ankle support that absorb the impact of your feet on the ground.

▶ Many women find swimming more pleasant and useful, because it puts less pressure on the spine, which does not have to support the weight of the body. It is important to swim without a board, because such a device could cause the back to arch, and also it is better to avoid swimming "frog-style," which could create problems for the spinal column. A swimming pool can be a source of infection, which is why it is a good general rule to pay particular at-

EXERCISE #1, LEVEL A

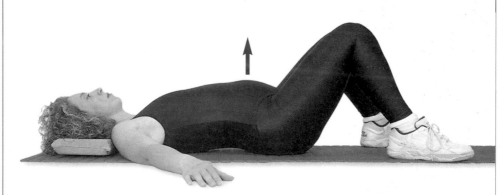

Lie on your back, knees bent, arms relaxed, feet firmly on the floor. Inhale; then, as you exhale, contract your abdominal muscles, flattening the small of your back and slightly raising the pubic area. Hold this position as you exhale. Inhale, relax, and repeat.

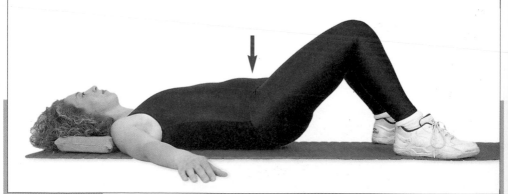

tention to the cleanliness of the area and to your own personal hygiene.

▶ From the fourth month on, exercises you do while lying on your back could create problems. This is because the baby presses on the inferior vena cava, which allows blood to flow to the heart. It is best to change the position to sitting or standing, or place a folded cloth under one hip so as to shift the baby and make the exercise easier to do.

More suitable exercises at that time in your pregnancy (after the 4th month) are **breathing exercises** (see page 38); **cervical, thoracic, lumbar, and overall spinal mobility exercises** (see pages 39 to 41 and 43 to 45); **stretching exercises** (see page 46); and **Level A exercises**, especially numbers **1, 3, 8,** and **10** (see below). Walking and swimming are recommended for warmups because the specific warmup workout suggested in this text can overstimulate the spine during pregnancy, particularly the lumbar region, with annoying consequences, especially as your weight increases.

EXERCISE #3, LEVEL A

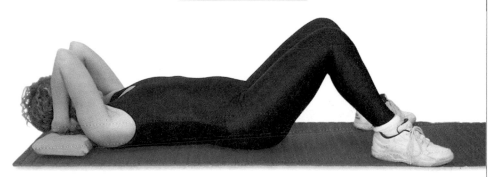

Lie on your back, knees bent, feet firmly on the floor, hands behind your head, elbows close together. Inhale; exhale and, using your arms to help you, lift head and shoulders from the floor without arching your back. Inhale, relax, and repeat.

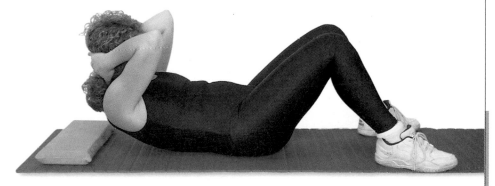

POSTPARTUM
(AFTER CHILDBIRTH)

During pregnancy, a woman undergoes changes from both the physical and psychological points of view. Immediately following childbirth, other factors appear, which cause a certain changeability, factors which should be considered if a woman wants to regain the equilibrium she had before.

From a physical point of view, the pelvis has widened in order to expel the baby during delivery, thanks to some hormones (progesterone and relaxin) that soften the tissues to permit a gradual relaxation of the body ligaments. The first consequence of this is a change in posture, with a heavy load at the lumbar level.

Other changes take place in the uterus, in the pelvic floor, and especially in the abdominal muscles. The first tangible effect following delivery is in the abdominal musculature, which appears flabby and lacking consistency, even though flatter than before. During pregnancy these muscles were stretched around the uterus and,

EXERCISE #8, LEVEL A (DURING PREGNANCY)

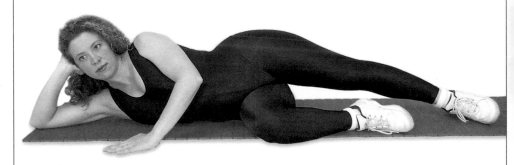

Lie on your right side, head resting on your right hand, right elbow on the floor, right knee bent, right leg in front of body, left leg extended to floor. Inhale; exhale, lifting left leg in line with upper body. Inhale, relax, and repeat. Do 6 repetitions; then change to left side.

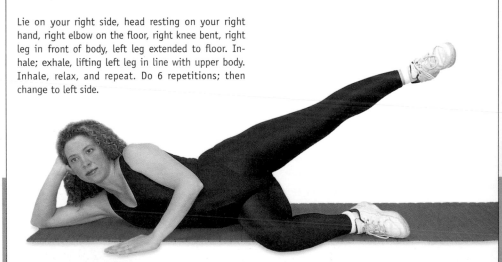

to return them to their original state, they need help and stimulation. The abdominal muscles are connected along the midline by a band of fibrous tissue called the linea alba (white line) which, thanks to the above-mentioned hormones, softens, permitting the two rectus abdominis muscles to stretch away from the midline, causing a weakening of the abdominal wall and the onset of lower back pain. This situation is aggravated in cases of multiple births, because the muscles are that much more strained and therefore they are even more in need of help.

When the abdominal musculature does not provide proper support to the bowels and internal organs, it causes constipation, a condition already in existence because of intestinal lethargy created by the action of progesterone and relaxin.

All these considerations, along with those of an emotional and psychological nature, lead to the urgency to start working out within the first 48 hours following delivery, while still in the hospital, even though this might seem strange.

EXERCISE #10, LEVEL A (DURING PREGNANCY)

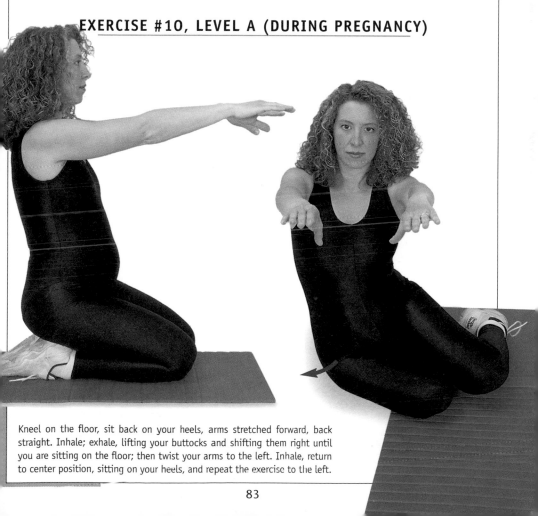

Kneel on the floor, sit back on your heels, arms stretched forward, back straight. Inhale; exhale, lifting your buttocks and shifting them right until you are sitting on the floor; then twist your arms to the left. Inhale, return to center position, sitting on your heels, and repeat the exercise to the left.

83

Postpartum exercises

The same instructions given for work on the abdominal muscles under normal conditions apply to performing the exercises postpartum, and they are:
- Do not push exercise to the point of fatigue or strain;
- Stop if your body sends out warning signals (nausea, dizziness);
- Listen to your body and to the feelings it is sending;
- Find the most appropriate time to work out.

▶ Self-evaluation of your abdominal muscles

You can evaluate the condition of your abdominal muscles before starting a workout, using the space between the rectus abdominis muscles as a reference point. Lie on your back, knees bent, one arm at your side, the other hand on your stomach. Raise your head and shoulders, reaching the outstretched arm towards your feet; with the other hand, feel the space between the two rectus abdominis muscle bands. At first this space may be 2 or 3 fingers wide; with time and training it may decrease, indicating improved muscle tone and a return to normal.

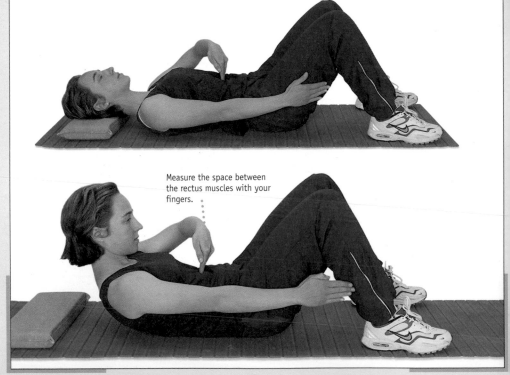

Measure the space between the rectus muscles with your fingers.

FIRST 48 HOURS POSTPARTUM AND FOR THE NEXT 6 WEEKS

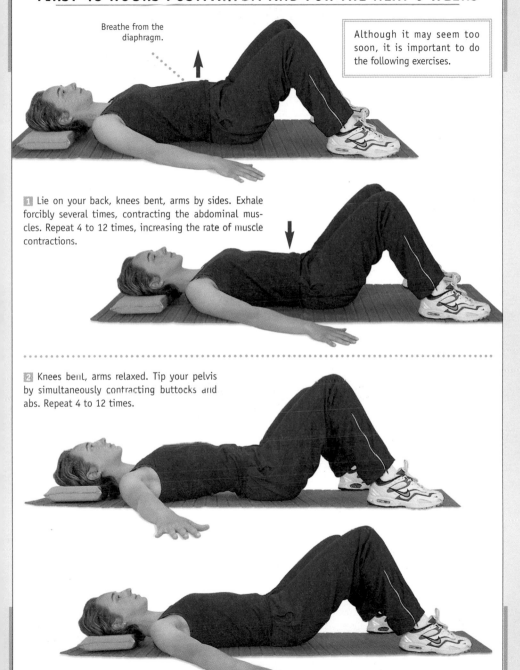

Breathe from the diaphragm.

Although it may seem too soon, it is important to do the following exercises.

1 Lie on your back, knees bent, arms by sides. Exhale forcibly several times, contracting the abdominal muscles. Repeat 4 to 12 times, increasing the rate of muscle contractions.

2 Knees bent, arms relaxed. Tip your pelvis by simultaneously contracting buttocks and abs. Repeat 4 to 12 times.

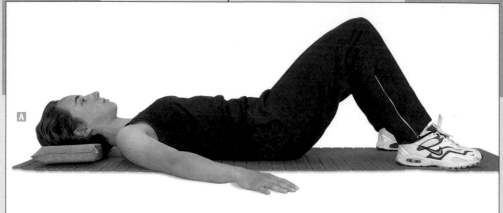

3 Knees bent, arms by your sides. Contracting the abs and buttocks to effect a pelvic tip, let your legs slide down and back, without arching your back. Repeat 4 to 12 times.

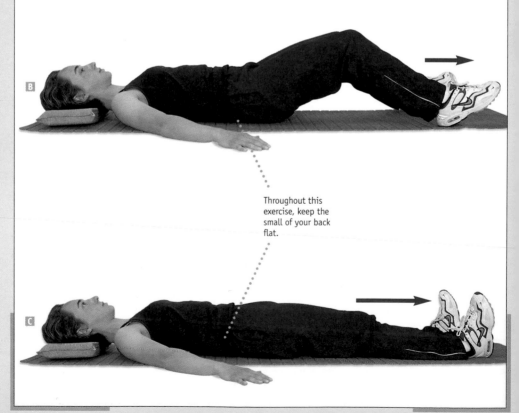

Throughout this exercise, keep the small of your back flat.

Breathing, relaxation, and upper body toning exercises will be added later to the exercises described here.

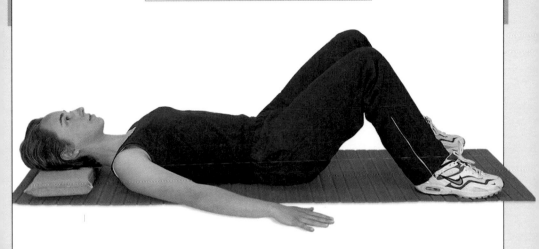

4 Knees bent, arms by your sides. Inhale; exhale, raising head, shoulders, and arms, reaching toward your feet. Hold this position as you count to four, then slowly lie back down. Repeat 4 to 8 times, increasing the hold time from 4 to 10 seconds.

Lift your head, shoulders, and arms in that order; reverse the order as you lie down.

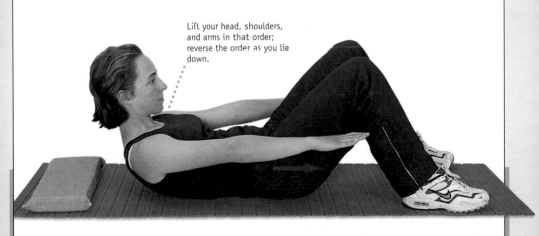

FROM 6 WEEKS TO 3 MONTHS POSTPARTUM

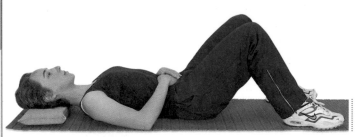

1 Lie on back, knees bent, hands on stomach. Inhale and, contracting the buttocks, raise upper body; exhale and, contracting your abs, raise head. Hold this position for 4 seconds. Increase hold time until you get to 10 seconds. Repeat 4 to 8 times.

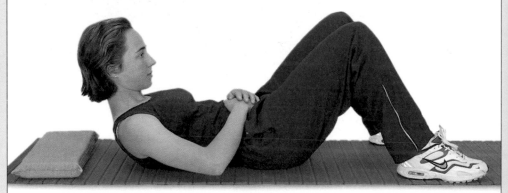

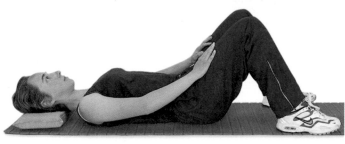

2 Lie on back, knees bent, hands on thighs. Inhale; exhale, raising head. Contract buttocks and abs, bringing hands to knees, and hold this position for 4 seconds. Repeat 5 to 10 times.

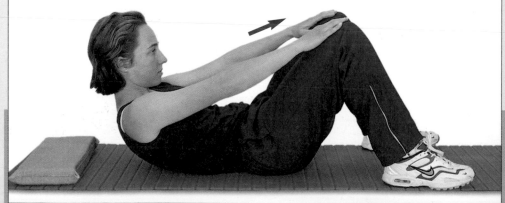

3 Lie on back, knees bent, arms by sides. Exhale and, reaching your right hand to your left foot, twist your torso. Lie back down and repeat on the other side. Repeat 5 to 20 times.

During the torso twist, always keep control of the cervical (neck) area.

4 Lie on your back, knees bent, arms by your sides. Exhale, raising head and shoulders and bringing your left hand to your left foot, keeping abs and buttocks contracted. Lie back down and repeat on the other side. Repeat 5 to 20 times.

5 Lie on right side, head resting on right hand, the other hand on the floor by your chest. Inhale; exhale, lifting your left leg out and up, and hold this position for 4 seconds. Repeat 5 to 20 times on each side, increasing the hold time from 4 to 10 seconds.

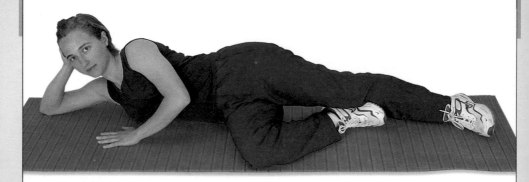

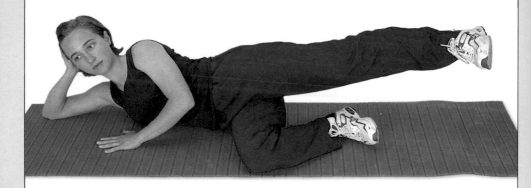

6 Sit on the floor, knees bent, hands on your stomach. Inhale; exhale, slowly leaning back toward the floor, and stop halfway down for 4 seconds. Repeat 5 to 10 times, increasing the hold time from 4 to 10 seconds.

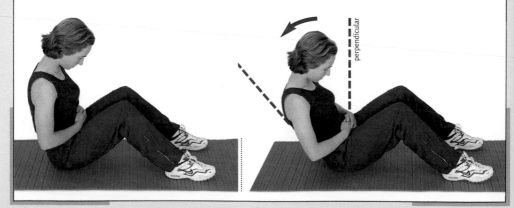

perpendicular

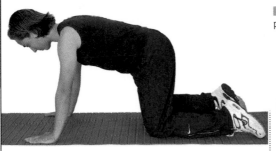

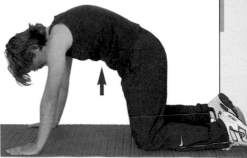

7 Get down on all fours, hands and knees supporting body weight as shown in left photo.

Exhale, contracting buttocks and abs and pushing your back upward. Inhale, returning to starting position. Repeat 10 to 20 times.

FROM 3 TO 6 MONTHS POSTPARTUM

1 Lie on your back, hands behind your head, knees bent toward chest. Inhale; exhale and, without lifting your shoulders off the floor, twist your bent knees to the right, keeping them raised. Return to the center position and repeat to the other side. Repeat 5 to 20 times.

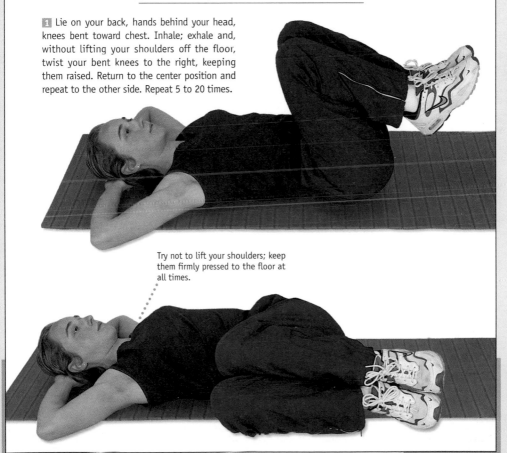

Try not to lift your shoulders; keep them firmly pressed to the floor at all times.

91

2 Sit on the floor, hands behind head, knees bent. Inhale; exhale, slowly leaning back towards the floor, and lower your lumbar area, chest, shoulders, and head in that order. Sit back up, using your arms to help you. Repeat 5 to 10 times.

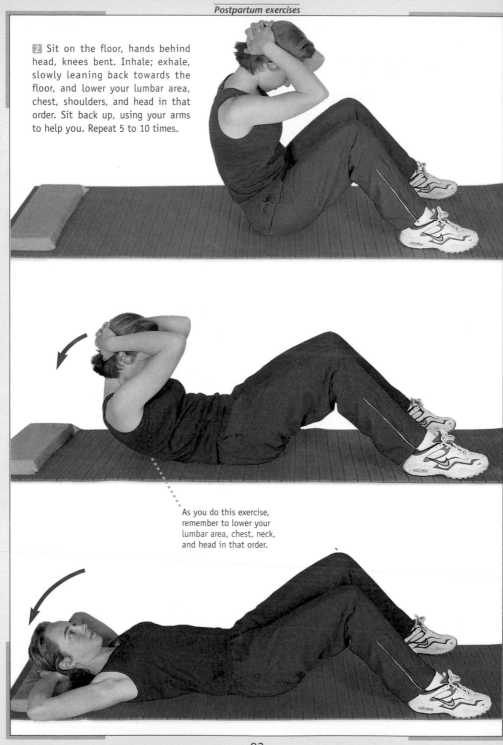

As you do this exercise, remember to lower your lumbar area, chest, neck, and head in that order.

3 Lie on your right side, legs outstretched, head resting in right hand, left hand on the floor in front of your chest. Inhale; exhale, raising both legs together; then lower them. Repeat 5 to 10 times.

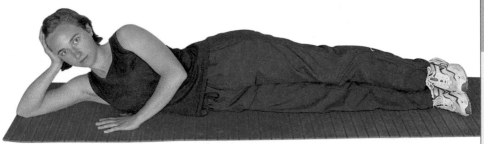

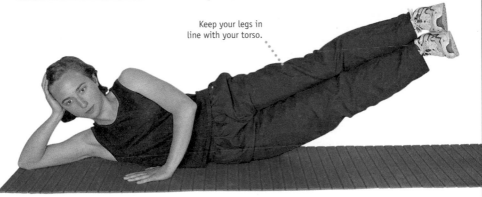

Keep your legs in line with your torso.

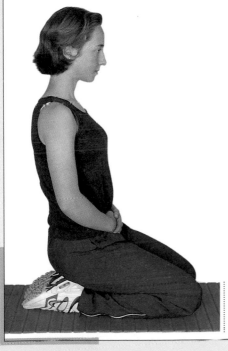

4 Kneel, hands on your stomach. Exhale, leaning backward, contracting buttocks and abs. Inhale, returning to start. Repeat this exercise 5 to 10 times.

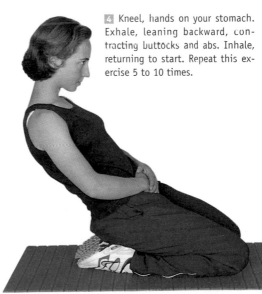

EQUIPMENT TO STRENGTHEN ABS

The industry for home exercise equipment is flourishing and frequently comes out with new equipment. This results from one very simple fact: even though the gym may be convenient, nearby, and open all hours of the day and maybe even at night, exercising at home is still more convenient. Nevertheless, let's remember that we must be filled with good will, constancy, and interest in the home workout we plan to undertake. The temptation to give up the activity is always lying in wait, with the inevitable consequence that the new equipment, purchased with so much enthusiasm, will end its days buried in dust in the cellar.

> Given the success of telemarketing, we cannot avoid mentioning a new piece of equipment, which produces electrostimulation of muscles, promising dazzling results. Electrostimulation is extremely useful in the functional rehabilitation of limbs afflicted with specific problems, but in any event should be used only under the strict supervision of competent personnel who can design progressive workout sessions tailored to the actual needs of the user.

▶ For this reason, it is extremely important to carefully evaluate the equipment we would like to buy and the goal we hope to reach.

If the goal is to improve cardiorespiratory capacity, it is not necessary to rush out and buy a computerized treadmill; a bicycle and some comfortable jogging outfits will do for starters.

If your objective is the well-being of your abs, buying cumbersome and costly equipment does not make much sense, especially if space is limited: it would be better to focus on a small piece of equipment or an abdominal bench. And if you are a fan of infomercials, be wary of anyone who promises that you can lose inches from your waist and get back to the shape you were in decades earlier very quickly and with no effort. Such miracles happen very rarely indeed!

▶ To help you in your selection, we have examined two pieces of equipment that are available on the market at modest prices: an ab roller and a decline abdominal bench.

I suggest not allotting more than half of your available workout time to equipment use; it's better to work out with your body alone, which will let you find a balance between body and mind more easily.

▶ Finally, we want to discredit the myth that clothing of plastic, neoprene, or similar materials let you sweat off excess pounds. This is in the realm of science fiction; the only thing that happens in reality is a steady loss of fluids, which hopefully are replaced when you drink water, but which at times can cause dehydration. Unfortunately, dehydration is typical of someone who trains by running covered in plastic, seeking that imaginary sense of well-being produced by a "good sweat."

Ab roller

The first device we looked at, an ab roller, can be very useful because, if used according to instructions, it prevents overstimulation of the cervical spine (neck), which can occur with exercises #3 and #4 of Level A. In cases of pain in the cervical area, an ab roller may allow you to do the workout you planned without foregoing a session. The recommended exercises follow.

EXERCISE #1

Head rests on the neck pad, feet firmly on floor, hands grip the upper part of handles. Inhale; exhale, raising your upper body to about a 45-degree angle, using the strength in your arms to help you. Inhale and relax. Repeat 10 times.

Do not strain your cervical area excessively.

EXERCISE #2

Head rests on the neck pad, feet firmly on floor, hands grip the upper part of the handles (see position on page 95). Inhale; exhale, raising your upper body about 45 degrees while at the same time lifting your feet from the floor and bringing your knees to your chest. Inhale and relax. Repeat 10 times.

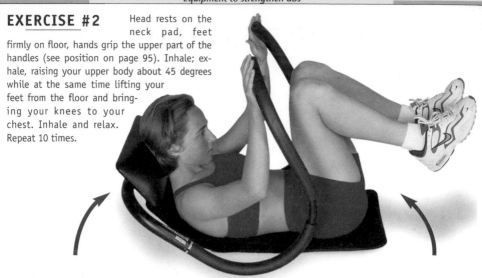

EXERCISE #3

Head rests on the neck pad, hands grip the upper part of handles. Knees bent to one side, feet off floor.

Inhale; exhale, raising your upper body about 45 degrees, keeping your knees immobile. Inhale, relax, and repeat the exercise, bending knees to the other side. Repeat 6 times per side.

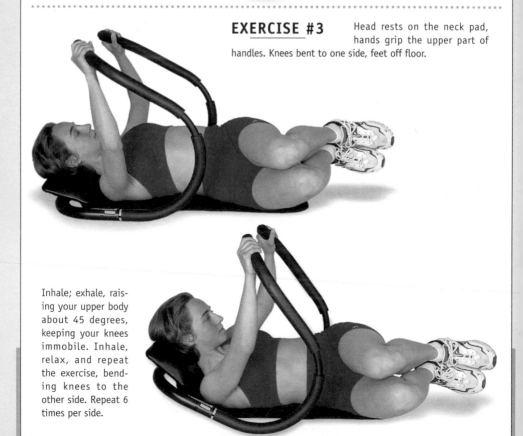

Decline ab bench

The decline abdominal bench allows us to get good results because it puts the abdominal muscle system to work at various angles. Exercises need to be done with control of the position of the lumbar area, keeping the back in proper alignment. Let's look at some useful exercises.

EXERCISE #1

Sit on bench, feet on the lower support, hands on stomach and head bent forward. Inhale; exhale, lowering your upper body about 15 to 20 degrees, and hold the position for 5 seconds.

Keep your head bent forward.

perpendicular

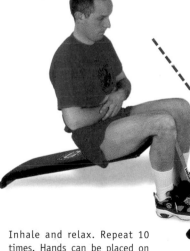

Inhale and relax. Repeat 10 times. Hands can be placed on chest or behind head, depending on your level of fitness.

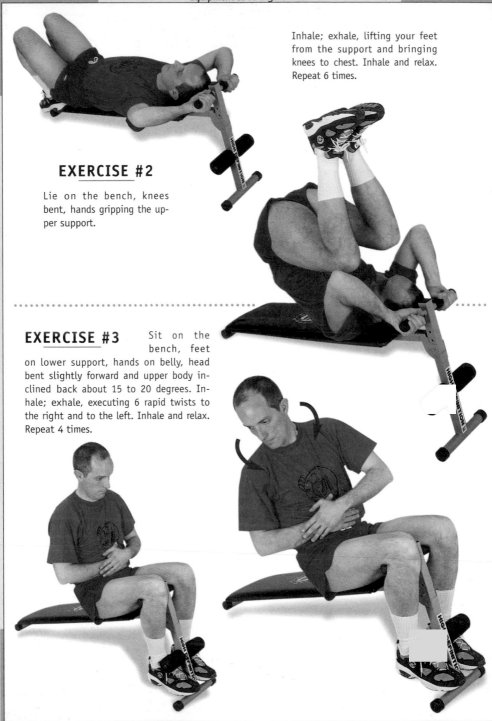

Inhale; exhale, lifting your feet from the support and bringing knees to chest. Inhale and relax. Repeat 6 times.

EXERCISE #2

Lie on the bench, knees bent, hands gripping the upper support.

EXERCISE #3

Sit on the bench, feet on lower support, hands on belly, head bent slightly forward and upper body inclined back about 15 to 20 degrees. Inhale; exhale, executing 6 rapid twists to the right and to the left. Inhale and relax. Repeat 4 times.

MUSCLES AND NUTRITION

As often mentioned, the idea that a single change can resolve all your body's problems is not realistic. In fact, drawing up a plan of action without taking nutrition into consideration, or else obsessing about weight, may be self-defeating.

Many times fitness mistakenly is equated with weight loss: "I am out of shape... I need to lose a few pounds!"

Many of the directions about nutrition have already been mentioned in the paragraph "Sources of energy for muscle work" (page 18). We will now examine these in depth.

We will give you suggestions designed to make a balanced diet part of the healthy habits of your everyday life.

We will suggest a sane, healthy, and easy-to-plan way of eating, without making sacrifices or suffering the discomforts typical of diets often published in newspapers or recommended by neighbors (yo-yo diets, vegetable soup diets, etc.).

A BALANCED DIET

A balanced diet includes a large variety of foods, which allow the body to grow and stay in good health by supplying energy to it. In order to survive, a person needs proteins, fats, carbohydrates, vitamins, minerals, fiber, and water. Consult a good nutrition book to learn more about the sources and uses of these nutrients and vitamins.

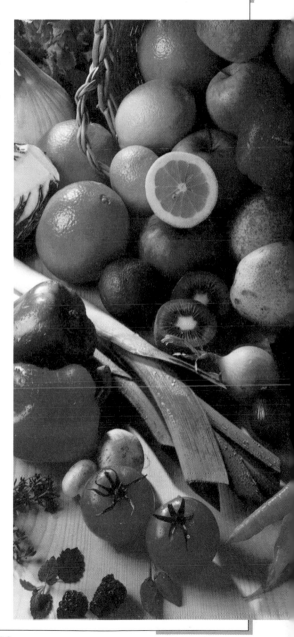

PROTEINS

In moderate amounts, proteins are essential, as they are used in the production of the cells of bodily tissues. Proteins also produce enzymes (substances which regulate cellular reaction), hormones, and important blood components. They can be found in **seafood**, **eggs**, **cereals**, **dairy products**, **nuts**, **legumes**, **and meat**. Proteins are made up of basic elements called amino acids. In the absence of other sources of energy, proteins are burned by the body (proteins supply 4 calories per gram).

CARBOHYDRATES

Carbohydrates are the principal and most effective source of energy for growth, sustenance, and bodily function. A meal should consist primarily of carbohydrates. They supply 4 calories of energy per gram. Carbohydrates can be found in many kinds of food: **bread**, **pasta**, **potatoes**, **rice**, **grains**, **fruit**, **and vegetables**. The principal kinds of carbohydrate are cellulose, starch, and sugar. Cellulose is not digested, but helps in the digestion of other foods. Excess carbohydrates are stored in the liver and muscles to be used when you fast or during physical exercise.

FATS

Like carbohydrates, fats are used by the body as a source of energy, but fats supply more energy per unit weight (9 calories per gram). Excess fats accumulate in the form of fatty tissue under the skin or around the organs. There are two principal kinds of fat: **saturated fats** from animal sources (such as meat and butter), and **unsaturated fats**, found in nuts and olive oil. Too much animal fat can speed the onset of heart disease.

VITAMINS

Because the body cannot produce the majority of the vitamins it needs, they have to be acquired from food. They are divided into two groups: those soluble in fat (**vitamins A, D, E, and K**) and those soluble in water (**vitamins C and B**). The former can be found in milk products, meat, eggs, and seafood. Vitamin A is important for vision, vitamin D for bones, and K for blood coagulation. Water-soluble vitamins can be found in vegetables and fruits, grains, meat, and poultry; they facilitate food assimilation.

MINERALS

The body does not produce any minerals, although they are needed to build bones, regulate fluid balance, control nerves and muscles, and produce energy. Correct mineral intake is helped by a very varied diet. The most important minerals, required in fairly high quantities, are: **calcium**, **potassium**, **sulfur**, **phosphorous**, **sodium**, **chlorine**, **iron**, **iodine**, and **magnesium**. Other minerals necessary, although in lesser quantities, are called secondary or trace minerals. Cauliflower, spinach, watercress, shrimp, lettuce, and lentils are rich in minerals.

FIBER

Most fiber is not assimilated by the body, but plays an important role in the digestion.

It makes the stool compact and soft so it can be easily eliminated, thus preventing certain intestinal disorders and the onset of constipation. According to some people, fiber can reduce the risk of getting certain diseases, including heart disease. The majority of fiber can be found in **fruit**, **vegetables**, **whole wheat bread**, and in the outer **coating of grains (bran, brown rice)**.

WATER

Drinking is very important, even more so than eating. In fact, though it is possible to survive without solid food for a long time, it is extremely dangerous to go without liquid intake even for a few days (liquids taken in as such or through food). The seriousness of this situation is aggravated when certain climate conditions exist, or in the presence of severe dehydration, which may be caused by a disease such as dysentery. As an adult loses on average **3 liters** (about 3 quarts) **of water a day** through sweat and excretion, it is essential to restore fluid balance to avoid a variety of problems, including constipation, skin problems, digestive disorders, and dehydration.

In a diet rich in fruit and fresh vegetables, water content is elevated about half a liter (16 oz) a day; the amount needed to reach 3 liters must be added by drinking.

WHAT HAPPENS WHEN WE EAT

When we ask someone what he or she eats every day, the most frequent answer is: "I eat normally! When I have time, a first course, a main course with side dishes, dessert, and coffee; if I can, some wine and an appetizer, otherwise a nice sandwich." Choosing what to eat is best done with some knowledge, so let's learn a little about digestion.

▶ Digestion starts in the mouth, assisted by chewing but mainly by saliva, which contains certain digestive enzymes (e.g., ptyalin), which begin the digestion of the complex carbohydrates (bread, pasta, rice).

▶ In the stomach, the chewed food or bolus is acted on by gastric juices, whose composition varies according to the food ingested.

▶ From the stomach, it passes through the pylorus into the intestine where bile, along with other pancreatic juices, completes the digestive process. At this point the fundamental nutrients are absorbed, move into the blood, and are carried to all organs of the body. Any unused material goes into the large intestine and is then eliminated. Fluids pass through the kidneys, where they are filtered, and waste then is expelled.

▶ From our analysis, we can see that eating different types of food, particularly in incorrect combinations, risks delaying digestion times, thus impeding absorption of basic nutrients. Let's take a look at a typical diet (ctd. on page 104).

COMPOSITION OF FOODS: WATER, PROTEIN, FATS
AND CARBOHYDRATES for each 100-gram serving (about 3.5 oz)

FOOD	WATER (grams)	PROTEIN (grams)	FATS (grams)	USABLE CARBOHYDRATES (grams)
CEREALS & GRAINS*				
wheat germ	10.0	28.0	10.0	55.0
corn	12.5	9.2	3.8	75.8
pearl barley	12.2	10.4	1.4	82.3
bread, Type 1	34.0	8.9	0.6	60.3
whole wheat bread	36.6	7.5	1.3	53.8
whole wheat flour	13.4	11.9	1.9	68.4
white flour, Type 0	14.2	11.5	1.0	76.9
white flour, Type 00	14.2	11.0	0.7	78.0
LEGUMES				
chick peas	13.0	21.8	4.9	54.3
beans (dry)	10.7	23.6	2.5	51.7
string beans (fresh)	90.5	2.1	0.1	2.4
shelled broad beans	13.3	27.2	3.0	55.3
lentils (dry)	11.6	25.0	2.5	54.0
peas (fresh)	76.1	7.4	0.2	12.4
GREENS & VEGETABLES				
red beets	91.3	1.1	0	4.0
artichokes	84.0	2.7	0.2	2.5
carrots	91.6	1.1	0	7.6
cauliflower	90.5	3.2	0.2	2.7
Brussels sprouts	85.7	4.2	0.5	4.3
onions	92.1	1.0	0.1	5.7
fennel	93.2	1.2	0	1.0
mushrooms	2.1	2.3	0.4	1.9
lettuce	94.3	1.8	0.4	2.2
potatoes	78.5	2.1	1.0	18.0
ripe tomatoes	94.0	1.0	0.2	3.5
leeks	87.8	2.1	0.1	5.2
parsley	87.2	3.7	0.6	trace
endives	88.1	1.9	0.5	0.5
radishes	95.6	0.8	0.1	1.8
celery	88.3	2.3	0.2	2.4
spinach	90.1	3.4	0.7	3.0
yellow squash	94.6	1.1	0.1	3.5
FRESH FRUIT				
apricots	86.3	0.4	0.1	6.8
pineapples	86.4	0.5	0	10.0

FOOD	WATER (grams)	PROTEIN (grams)	FATS (grams)	USABLE CARBOHYDRATES (grams)
oranges	87.2	0.7	0.2	7.8
bananas	79.8	1.2	0.3	15.5
chestnuts	41.0	3.5	1.8	42.4
figs	81.9	0.9	0.2	11.2
strawberries	90.5	0.9	0.4	5.3
lemons	89.5	0.6	0	2.3
apples	85.6	0.2	0.3	11.0
peaches	90.7	0.8	0.1	6.1
grapes	80.3	0.5	0.1	15.6
DRIED FRUIT & NUTS				
figs	19.4	3.5	2.7	66.6
hazelnuts	5.7	13.0	62.9	1.8
walnuts	6.3	15.8	63.7	6.3
green olives	76.8	0.8	15.0	1.0
plums	29.3	2.2	0.5	37.1
raisins	17.1	1.9	0.6	72.0
MEAT				
rabbit (semi-fat)	70.9	22.1	5.3	0.5
chicken (breast)	75.3	22.2	0.9	-
lean ham	54.8	28.6	11.5	0
turkey (breast)	70.2	22.0	6.2	0.4
SWEETS				
honey	18.0	0.6	0	80.3
sugar (sucrose)	0.5	0	0	104.5
FISH & SEAFOOD				
anchovies	76.5	16.8	2.6	1.5
codfish	81.5	17.0	0.3	-
sardines	73.0	20.8	4.5	(1.5)
sole	79.5	16.9	1.7	9.8
trout	80.5	14.7	3.0	-
MILK, CHEESE & EGGS				
cow's milk (whole)	87.0	3.1	3.4	4.8
cow's milk (skim)	90.5	3.6	0.2	5.3
Fontina cheese	41.1	24.5	26.9	0.8
Parmesan cheese	29.5	36.0	25.6	trace
Pecorino cheese	32.3	28.5	28.0	trace
chicken eggs (whites)	87.6	10.9	trace	0.8
chicken eggs (yolks)	49.2	16.3	31.9	0.7

Under "Usable Carbohydrates," simple sugars (those which commonly give a sweet flavor) are included. This is because, for example, red beets and carrots contain a certain amount of carbohydrates even though they are not starchy vegetables.
*Here we list the average composition of brown rice and whole wheat pasta. Brown rice: protein, 7.5 g; fat, 2.2 g; carbohydrates, 75.4 g. Whole wheat pasta: protein, 12.5 g; fat, 1.2 g; carbohydrates, 75 g.

If we start with a first course of pasta (complex carbohydrates), we see that this is attacked first by ptyalin and then by the gastric juices in the stomach, which proceed with digestion. You will notice that no mention was made of pasta with meat sauce, because that would complicate matters; you'll soon see why!

Now we move on to the main course, steak: the proteins it contains have completely opposite digestive requirements to those of the pasta. The steak is attacked in the mouth by pepsin and not ptyalin, and in the stomach by hydrochloric acid, creating an acidic environment that suspends the carbohydrate processing of the pasta. Until the meat passes through, the pasta stays where it is and the digestive process slows down.

As you can see, the job is getting complicated and it gets even more so when we move on to dessert (simple sugars). Sugars should go directly to the intestine to be absorbed at the gastric level, but, finding other food there, they are stopped and begin fermenting.

Things are definitely complicated, so why not resolve matters with a nice cup of coffee?

Coffee increases the already-existing acidity level and tries to mask the uncomfortable situation, a feeling of inertia, sleepiness, and digestive difficulty, by giving the nervous system a small jolt.

The above points out the errors in our normal eating patterns and opens a discussion on fitness weight, energy needs, and food combinations.

FITNESS WEIGHT OR OPTIMAL WEIGHT

Maintaining body weight is very important if we want to enjoy good health. This concept is often blurred with rivers of ink and words that only create confusion. To define fitness or optimal weight is not simple, but it could be described as that physical condition which gives each one of us the pleasant feeling of psychophysical well-being and fills us with vitality.

▶ Optimal body weight is theoretical and is very closely allied with personality type, since there are those who claim to feel good about themselves and their bodies despite obviously being overweight or underweight. To be more scientific and rational, you can find your own optimal body weight by making use of the chart on the facing page.

▶ If your actual weight is 20% or less above your optimal weight, it is classified as overweight. If the excess weight is greater than 20%, it is called obesity. Obesity is not only an esthetic problem, but unfortunately predisposes one to various illnesses, including hypertension, diabetes, and heart disease. Underweight can also be the source of problems, particularly in the young.

Body weight depends primarily on calories consumed in proportion to activities performed. In general, weight is kept stable if the number of calories taken in and the number of calories used are equal. Even small excesses can cause significant changes in the long term.

ENERGY NEEDS

Energy needs can be divided into two parts: the energy necessary to maintain basal metabolism (the expenditure of energy the body needs during conditions of minimal physical and mental activity) and the energy necessary to perform specific activities.

EVALUATING YOUR BODY WEIGHT

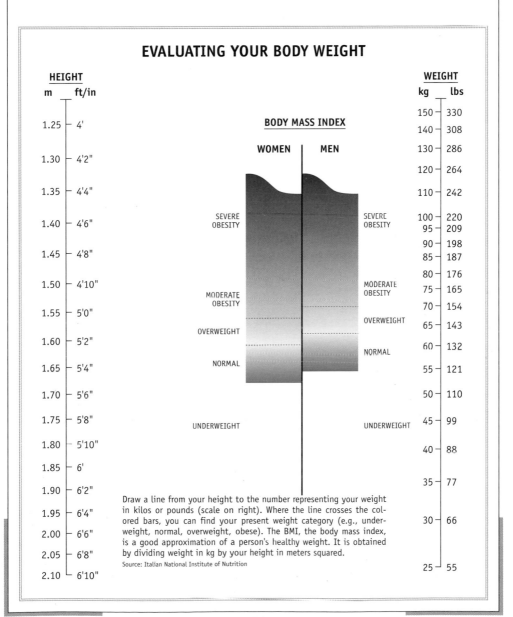

HEIGHT
m   ft/in

WEIGHT
kg   lbs

BODY MASS INDEX

WOMEN   MEN

1.25 — 4'	150 — 330
	140 — 308
1.30 — 4'2"	130 — 286
	120 — 264
1.35 — 4'4"	110 — 242
1.40 — 4'6"	100 — 220
	95 — 209
1.45 — 4'8"	90 — 198
	85 — 187
1.50 — 4'10"	80 — 176
	75 — 165
1.55 — 5'0"	70 — 154
1.60 — 5'2"	65 — 143
	60 — 132
1.65 — 5'4"	55 — 121
1.70 — 5'6"	50 — 110
1.75 — 5'8"	45 — 99
1.80 — 5'10"	40 — 88
1.85 — 6'	
1.90 — 6'2"	35 — 77
1.95 — 6'4"	
2.00 — 6'6"	30 — 66
2.05 — 6'8"	
2.10 — 6'10"	25 — 55

SEVERE OBESITY

MODERATE OBESITY

OVERWEIGHT

NORMAL

UNDERWEIGHT

SEVERE OBESITY

MODERATE OBESITY

OVERWEIGHT

NORMAL

UNDERWEIGHT

Draw a line from your height to the number representing your weight in kilos or pounds (scale on right). Where the line crosses the colored bars, you can find your present weight category (e.g., underweight, normal, overweight, obese). The BMI, the body mass index, is a good approximation of a person's healthy weight. It is obtained by dividing weight in kg by your height in meters squared.

Source: Italian National Institute of Nutrition

Energy needs vary according to a person's age, gender, physical constitution, physical activity, and special situations such as pregnancy, nursing, and menopause. Considering that over the past ten years the average daily food consumption has increased far beyond recommended levels in many countries, it is important to remember that energy intake should be allocated as follows: 60% from carbohydrates; 30% fats; 10% proteins.

▶ The **food pyramid** (above) shows what proportion to allot to each food group that is in the daily diet.

▶ The table on pages 102 to 103 may be useful in choosing among the various foods and in staying on track with a balanced diet.

FOOD COMBINATIONS

It is useless to choose nourishing foods if they are not combined correctly. The wrong combination of foods alters the digestive process, weighing us down and thus "poisoning" our bodies, while the proper combination prevents these problems. Here are some things to avoid.

FATS SWEETS

MILK YOGURT **MEAT POULTRY SEAFOOD LEGUMES**

FRUIT **VEGETABLES**

BREAD CEREALS RICE

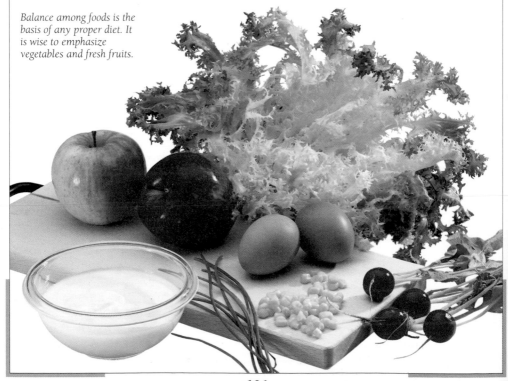

Balance among foods is the basis of any proper diet. It is wise to emphasize vegetables and fresh fruits.

BASIC IDEAS FOR PROPER NUTRITION

Before concluding, let's remember a few basic concepts:
- ▶ Eat regular meals (breakfast, lunch, dinner)
- ▶ Avoid eating between meals as much as possible
- ▶ Eat slowly
- ▶ Don't overdo alcoholic beverages
- ▶ Eat in moderation
- ▶ Don't give in to the temptations from your taste buds, and if you do, don't overindulge
- ▶ Drink a lot of water throughout the day
- ▶ Add fiber to your diet
- ▶ Don't skip meals

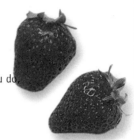

COMBINATIONS TO AVOID

▶ **Starchy foods with proteins.** Digestion of starches that have been cooked (e.g., pasta, rice, bread) starts in the mouth with ptyalin which, in order to accomplish this, is produced in great quantity. Production of hydrochloric acid in the stomach is inhibited to permit the ptyalin to continue the digestive process. If meat is added, digestion of starches is blocked, since they absorb the gastric juices needed to digest the meat.

▶ **Different proteins**. It is important to avoid combining meat and milk. In fact, in the stomach milk forms clots which surround the meat, keeping the gastric juices from carrying on the digestive process, which can resume only after the milk has curdled.

▶ **Food rich in simple sugars plus proteins and starches**. Simple sugars (candy, fruit, jam) if eaten between meals can easily be digested, but if eaten following a big meal consisting mainly of starches and meat, they can begin fermenting.

▶ **Fats and proteins**. Fats do not help gastric secretion, therefore it is not appropriate to combine cheese with meat, or butter and cream with vegetables or fried food, because digestion will be retarded.

CORRECT COMBINATIONS

There are foods which can be combined without fear of indigestion. They are:

- Pasta and vegetables
- Legumes and vegetables
- Meat and vegetables
- Cheese and vegetables
- Fruit and sweets
- Bread and olives
- Bread and fleshy fruit
- Milk and acidic fruit
- Yogurt and acidic fruit

▶ Having already undergone preliminary digestion as a result of rising, **bread** – unlike pasta – can be combined with cheese, meat, and protein-rich foods in general.

Based on the instructions provided, or from your own research, try to design the diet best suited to you, one that will allow you to reach your goals. Always strive for the proper balance between what you eat and what you burn up, without imposing harsh restrictions on yourself; the aim is merely to find the best possible nutritional plan for yourself.

Afterword

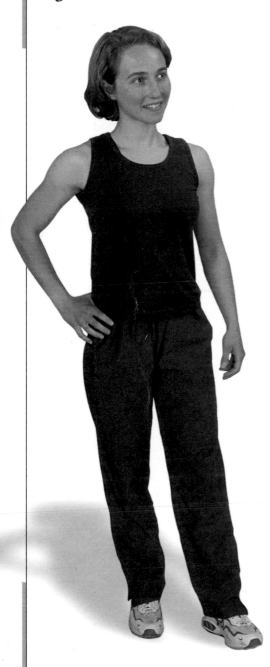

This book makes no pretense of fully covering all possible exercises for the abdominal musculature, but it does represent a starting point for focusing your attention on the needs of your body and seeking physical and mental well-being.

By going to the gym, using exercise equipment at home, or doing further research in other books, you can pursue a program that will help you improve your outward appearance and, above all, help you to do profound work on yourself with respect to your biorhythms and needs. The workout program you're about to embark on should be based on your own personal requirements and not on suggestions you might get from friends or fashion magazines.

Enjoy your workout!

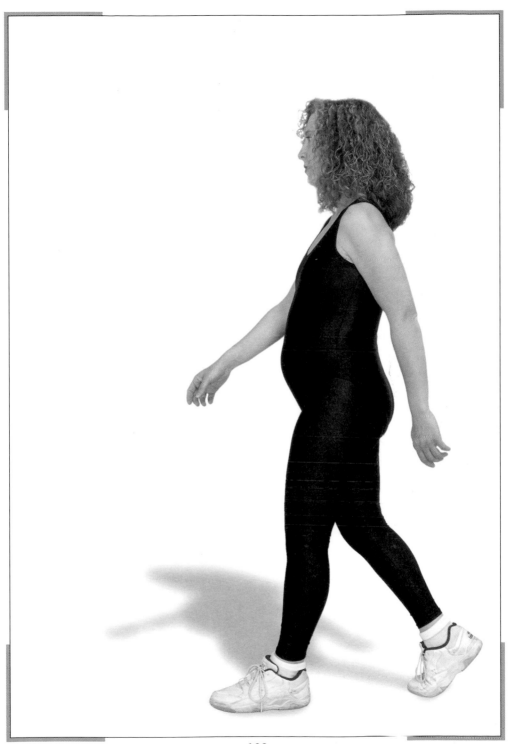

Index